# Participatory Video

Video can be a powerful tool for the self-expression and interaction in group development work. Used in a participatory way, video encourages people to examine the world around them, raising awareness of th on and helping them to become more actively involved in the decis ffect their lives. Based on an innovative approach researched over ars, *Participatory Video* offers a comprehensive guide to video work with groups, describing how to develop participants' abilities by involving them in using video creatively to record each other and their environment and tell their own stories.

The book includes over 60 step-by-step exercises, explaining clearly the procedure to follow, the time needed and the value of each activity. It provides basic information about video equipment and how to operate it, techniques for teaching production skills to group members and advice on planning, organizing and running a series of workshops and longer-term video projects. Jackie Shaw and Clive Robertson place the use of video within a coherent theoretical framework and show how to maximize its effectiveness in groups with a range of different needs.

*Participatory Video* will be of particular interest to group leaders looking for new ways to enhance and amplify the group development process. It is aimed at a wide range of professionals, including social workers, youth and community workers, teachers, probation officers, development educationalists, extension workers, therapists, community artists and video trainers.

**Jackie Shaw** and **Clive Robertson** are co-directors of Real Time Video, an educational charity specializing in developing group empowerment and self-advocacy through the use of video.

# Participatory Video

## A practical approach to using video creatively in group development work

■ Jackie Shaw and Clive Robertson

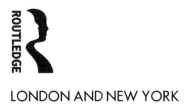

LONDON AND NEW YORK

First published 1997
by Routledge
11 New Fetter Lane, London EC4P 4EE

Simultaneously published in the USA
and Canada
by Routledge
29 West 35th Street, New York, NY 10001

© 1997 Jackie Shaw and Clive Robertson

Typeset in Times and Futura by
Solidus (Bristol) Limited
Printed and bound in Great Britain by
Redwood Books, Trowbridge, Wiltshire

*British Library Cataloguing in Publication
Data*

A catalogue record for this book is available
from the British Library

*Library of Congress Cataloguing in
Publication Data*

Shaw, Jackie
    Participatory video : a practical approach
    to using video creatively in group
    development work / Jackie Shaw and
    Clive Robertson.
    Includes bibliographical references and
    index.
    1.  Social group work.   2.  Video
    recording in social service.
    I.  Robertson, Clive      II.  Title.
    HV45.S47                          1997
    361.4 '028–dc20              96–36349

ISBN  0-415-14104-4
ISBN  0-415-14105-2 (pbk)

*Dedicated to*
*Essie Robertson*
*and the memory of*
*Janet Shaw*

# Contents

# Figures

# Preface

This book has grown out of our experience using video as a group development tool over the last twelve years. We began organizing video projects whilst working on an arts project for young people in the early 1980s. Excited by video's potential as a catalyst for participatory education and community action, we founded Real Time Video, an educational charity specializing in the creative use of video for group empowerment and self-advocacy.

Since then we have researched and developed a comprehensive approach through working with a wide range of people, including people with physical and learning disabilities, young people, older people, women, Black people, people recovering from mental ill-health, unemployed people, tenants, homeless people, and with many community-based groups and non-governmental organizations (NGOs) in the UK and overseas.

Video equipment is increasingly affordable and available. Most groups can gain access to a camcorder, but video's potential as a tool for group development is rarely fully exploited because there is a lack of knowledge about how to use it successfully.

From the mid-1980s we have been running training courses for other professionals wanting to use video effectively in their work. *Participatory Video* has resulted from the expressed need of group work facilitators from a variety of disciplines for a practical guide to this application of video.

# Acknowledgements

The photographs were taken by Ken Dickinson, the illustrations drawn by Larry Watson and the cover designed from an original idea by Tony Fox. Thanks to Nigel Bish, Anne-Marie Carty, Hur Ben Corrêa da Silva, Tony Dowmunt, Marie Groucott, Alison Haymonds and Donna Strough for all the help with the manuscript.

Thanks also to Marion Berry, Chris Blythe, Andrew Breary, Linda Chandler, Matthew Farrell, Pat Jennings, Debbi O'Brien, Mandy Parsons, Sue Smith, Larry Watson and Helen Wright at Real Time; to Shagufta Ali, Nick Ashwell, Mark Barratt, Tammy Bedford, Tim Bennett-Goodman, Guy Bentham, Paul Bramwell, Rosemary Brown, Steve Carpenter, Gabriel Chanan, Di Cook, Cathy Coulter, Bob Edwards, Gill Flanagan, Jane Gerson, Andrew Harland, Angela Hicks, Alan Jenkins, Keith Langton, Martin Mikhael, Pat Norrish, Kate Pestille, Monica Pinnock, Hazel Reed, Clive Ridgewell, Jayn Ritchie, Dave Richards, Kevin Shaw, Michael Thompson, Ruth Townsend and Liz Wheeler for advice and support; to Stephanie O'Connell, Acorn Resource Centre, Fairview Women's Open House, Lower Earley Lunch Club, Our Time, Reading Education and Training Centre, St Joseph's School and Woodley Hill House Black Students' Support Group for appearing in the photographs; to Reading Borough Council and Southern Arts for continued support and to all the people we've worked with over the years.

# Introduction

Participatory video is a group-based activity that develops participants' abilities by involving them in using video equipment creatively, to record themselves and the world around them, and to produce their own videos. In the communications age, where a constant stream of visual information is generated, over which most of the population have little control, using video can be a particularly pertinent way of shifting the balance of power and of opening up channels of communication for marginalized people.

There are currently significant changes taking place in society as a whole. Disintegration of traditional support networks and the resulting increased isolation and insecurity are affecting those least able to cope. Reorganization in many fields of work is resulting in fragmentation of services, yet this is accompanied by a desire for greater accountability and more user participation in choices affecting service provision. Organizations working in development worldwide are looking for ways to empower communities to express their needs and tell their own stories.

The participatory video approach can be an effective way of engaging people in the decisions that affect them, by developing their capacities and potential and by supporting the transfer of responsibility to them to enable them to voice their opinions and make real choices.

*Participatory Video* is written for group leaders looking for new ways to enhance and amplify the group development process. It is aimed at the wide variety of professionals involved in group work, including social workers, youth and community workers, teachers, development educationalists, extension workers, therapists, community artists, drama workers and video trainers.

The book guides the reader step by step through all aspects of participatory video work, covering theory and practice, as well as project management and equipment operation. It defines a clearly structured process, applicable to a broad range of situations, in an accessible, user-friendly style, and illustrates theory through exercises and project examples.

Following the suggested procedure will enable you to maximize the benefits of using video to develop participation, individual growth, communication, social cohesion, critical awareness, representation and self-determination.

## Using the book

*Participatory Video* is divided into the following four sections.

*Contexts* outlines the background to participatory video work in order to explore video's potential as a tool for group development and to clarify the motivations behind the approach.

*Workshops* covers the practicalities of running a video session, describing precisely what to do with the equipment in a group environment, and explaining why particular techniques are recommended to aid understanding. It outlines games and exercises to employ at each stage of the process, as well as general working practices to use in all the practical work.

*Projects* compares participatory video to other fields of work to look at possible applications. It expands on the benefits of longer-term video work, and explores how to set aims. It then describes how to organize a video project successfully, and how to plan a series of workshops tailored to a specific group.

*Equipment* covers the basic operational techniques needed to use video with groups, as well as how to teach technical skills to others.

The development of the participatory video approach throughout the book is not strictly linear because familiarity with the basic concepts explored in each of the four sections is required for full comprehension. For example, although *Projects* contains important overall perspectives, and much practical information that will be helpful before any face-to-face work begins, *Workshops* precedes *Projects* because some grasp of the nature of the actual workshop practice is necessary before considering more general project issues.

You are therefore advised to look at the four sections initially from start to finish, although it is not envisaged that the book will be used in a rigid cover-to-cover way. For instance, the *Workshops* section, particularly Chapter 3, contains much operational detail not needed until practical sessions start. After gaining some appreciation of the basic ideas presented in these chapters you may want to skim through the games and exercises on first reading. Later you can return to the particulars when browsing through the book to plan workshop sessions, or dip in and out of the chapters as necessary.

The book is structured for ease of use. Exercises are laid out consistently, making them straightforward to follow, and are self-contained so they can be used directly off the page. There are checklists at the end of each chapter to assist revision and assimilation, and operational and technical instructions are cross-referenced throughout.

Participatory video work requires a combination of skills, both technical and group work based. It is expected that most readers will have some knowledge and experience of working with people in groups, but a thorough explanation of the group work practice is included. If you are new to group development work, especially if you come from a technical background or have no experience of enabling other people, you are advised to gain some direct experience of the group work process by initially working alongside a more experienced facilitator.

No knowledge of video production is assumed but it is important that you practise operational techniques until you are confident before working with a group. All technical information is explained in non-jargonistic language, and technical instructions are separated from organizational procedure, so that the flow of the text is not interrupted by continual repetition. If you are new to video, work through the equipment section with reference to your video equipment, or refer to techniques and procedures as you come across them. If you have used video before, you are still advised to look through the technical section to make sure you understand how the equipment is utilized in participatory video work, in particular the strategies used to pass video skills on to other people effectively.

Video technology is developing fast. Newly available digital recording equipment, combined with the continued expansion in non-linear, computer-based editing, is certain to revolutionize video production capabilities in the late 1990s. *Participatory Video* has been written to take account of the changing nature of the medium. It concentrates on straightforward techniques that can produce results with video simply and quickly with a minimum of resources. As far as possible the technical sections present basic principles that are not equipment-specific, so that whatever technological advances are made in the future, the general procedures and group work practice will remain relevant and applicable.

The overall aim is to provide a clear guide to participatory video work. The intention is not to suggest that there is only one way of working with video, but for the sake of clarity a structured procedure has been distilled from what is essentially a complex multifaceted process. The resulting methodology is based on a wealth of practical experience. While constraints on book size prevented the inclusion of more real examples to illustrate points made, working practices and the reasoning behind them are always covered simultaneously. This will enable you to consider why a particular recommendation is appropriate and thus apply the approach flexibly to your own situation.

# Contexts

# Chapter 1

# Background, approach and benefits

## HISTORY

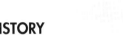

Video as a portable audio-visual recording medium has progressed rapidly since the first black-and-white reel-to-reel equipment became available in the mid-1960s. As the technology has developed, video's increasing adaptability and accessibility has resulted in a parallel growth in its application in a range of disciplines.

The use of video can be divided into three areas of activity: video in broadcasting, video as a domestic recording medium and video as a creative production medium (Armes 1988: 82–6, 128–30).

Following the development by Ampex of a 5cm (2in) broadcast-standard recorder in 1956, video has been used in broadcasting to preserve programme material. Previously television had been a predominantly live transmission medium, characterized by the absence of a satisfactory means of recording. Video has enabled programmes to be turned into lasting products that can be re-used internally, or packaged and sold to other consumers in the domestic market and overseas. In fact, most television is now recorded live within a studio setting and then transmitted from video at a later date.

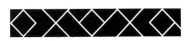

As portable broadcast-standard video systems have been devised, such as Betacam SP, video has also become the cheapest and most convenient way of recording news and location current affairs, and although the change has been slower, documentaries and dramatic productions are increasingly being recorded on video rather than film.

The second application of video has resulted from the availability of home video cassette recorders (VCRs) from the late 1970s onwards. Using much smaller 12mm (½in) tape, they were initially used to record broadcast programmes off-air to watch at leisure. Soon the replay potential was further exploited through the hire and sale of copies of films on video. This heralded widespread domestic use of the medium, and a mass market that ensured the commercial viability of continued research into technical improvements and new formats.

The other main area of video use is as a non-broadcast production medium. The black-and-white reel-to-reel Sony Rover, launched in 1965, was the first portable video production system. At that time heavy industrial machines were used in television, so its arrival was a major breakthrough, opening up the potential for non-broadcast video production. The introduction of the 20mm (¾in) U-Matic format in 1970, and the following development of editing recorders and battery-powered cameras, meant that this promise could be realized. The next twenty years saw an enormous expansion in non-broadcast users, and a plethora of new formats, driven by the quest for broadcast-standard portable systems on the one hand, and the growing domestic and non-broadcast professional markets on the other.

The greatest use of video as a production medium has been in the commercial sector, where companies have applied it extensively to promote their products and in training. Its use in pop videos has also made a significant impact.

Through the 1980s and into the 1990s, as prices have dropped and equipment has become smaller and lighter, there has also been an explosion in camcorder ownership. Video quickly replaced 8mm (5/16in) film as the amateur hobbyist format and now supplements photographs as a means of recording holidays and important personal events.

Video's evolution, as with all the preceding sound and image recording media, has been profit-led, motivated by commercial interest in mass reproduction and distribution.

> The ideal pattern would seem to be a three-fold pattern of profits (from the sale of a consumer durable, pre-recorded products, and recording materials): the triple market created at the turn of the century for cameras, postcards, and photographic materials is echoed in the 1980s by the combination of domestic video recorders, taped movies, and blank cassettes.

(Armes 1988: 113)

Nevertheless, video's potential as a social and creative tool was recognized early on, and non-profit applications were widely explored. Community workers, social workers, community arts workers and educationalists investigated its promise as a tool for social action and education; artists experimented with it as a creative medium; and independent video workers and community activists welcomed it as a way of democratizing access to the media. Throughout the late 1970s and early 1980s a vibrant independent video sector flourished in the UK, and a network of video organizations was established through a combination of local government, regional arts, and film and television funding.

Independent video is in this sense a very broad church. It includes most non-commercial, non-broadcast video production and distribution. The term implies an independence from commercial, governmental, broadcast network and mass audience concerns and control; from traditional modes of production and distribution; as well as from constraints on programme style and structure.

There is, of course, an inevitable overlap between the independent and the commercial and broadcast sectors. Independent tapes are sold for profit; tapes made about social issues, using new production processes, are broadcast; and the form of television is influenced by experimentation in the independent sector.

## VIDEO AND SOCIAL ACTION

Much work in the independent video sector is socially based. It is concerned with utilizing video as a tool for education and community action, and creating opportunities for under-represented groups to express their point of view. However, the work is not homogeneous. Within this area of video usage there is a range of approaches and widely differing opinion on the processes used. These different attitudes to non-broadcast social and community-based video work result in six areas of activity, outlined below.

### Production for the community

Production for the community is undertaken by video production units. They are set up to make tapes for under-represented sections of the community, and about social or educational issues that do not receive mass media coverage. Video units serve a range of groups, or a particular sector of the wider community, such as women or Black people.

Although this work can cover non-mainstream issues, it operates within a traditional television production model. A crew from the unit makes a programme for and about the community, and does not teach production skills to the people concerned.

## Provision of training and facilities

This area of activity aims to increase access to video production by providing affordable and accessible training courses and subsidized production and editing facilities. The aim is to enable groups and individuals to make their own programmes.

Courses cover all aspects of the production process at basic, intermediate and advanced levels. Some of them are targeted to increase usage by under-represented sections of the community, although attendance tends to be by the more self-assured and articulate members of those groups, who have the confidence to attend or the awareness that they have something to say.

## Exhibition and distribution

This work aims to create an audience for tapes made in the independent sector. Video programmes are distributed to community and educational groups through sales and hire services. They are then shown to an audience by a group leader who brings people together specifically to watch the tape, or at an event called a video screening.

Many tapes produced in this sector are designed to be discussion starters and to stimulate participation by the audience. They can be distributed with accompanying information detailing how to use them effectively.

Sometimes broadcast outlets are also developed. Videos made locally are shown on cable networks, and issue-based programmes fill access slots on television.

## Media education

This area of activity uses video as a tool to teach about the media in general and television in particular.

Much media education work explores television by deconstruction, breaking a programme into its component images and sounds, and analysing how the message is put together. Through using video, groups gain experience of constructing their own communications and this increases their understanding of the media.

Media education with video takes place in schools and colleges, and as part of some training courses provided for the community.

## Use of video in feedback

This application of video makes use of its immediate playback function. A particular activity or interaction is recorded; this can be an activity that would be taking place anyway but is often one set up specifically for the purpose of the exercise. The tape is then watched so that those taking part can learn from it.

Video feedback is used in the training of teachers, group leaders, counsellors and those who deal with the media. It is used to document social processes for research. Additionally it is used to provide behavioural, role-playing and communication skills feedback in social work and therapy, where it aims to help people change through a process of self-analysis.

## Participatory video

Participatory video work utilizes video as a social and community-based tool for individual and group development. Used in this way, video can be a powerful aid in the cultivation and realization of people's abilities and potential.

It is a group-based activity that revolves around the needs of the participants. Video is used to develop their confidence and self-esteem, to encourage them to express themselves creatively, to develop a critical awareness and to provide a means for them to communicate with others.

Participatory video is predominantly used with those disadvantaged by physical, attitudinal, educational, social or economic reasons, who would not usually express themselves through video, or attend a training course.

Active participation is an essential component. Group members operate the equipment for themselves, and a primary objective is the development of their control over their own work.

These different areas of video work all seek to exploit the potential of video as a social and educational tool. Although there can clearly be some overlap in activity, each type of video work has intrinsically different objectives. This affects the specific emphasis in every aspect of the work, the goals set, and the consequent outcomes.

This book concentrates on participatory video as a distinct discipline in order to explore in detail the aims of the approach, the working practices, and how it can be applied in a variety of settings.

## PARTICIPATORY VIDEO

The fundamental objective of participatory video work is to create a climate that encourages individual and group development. The specific technical and organizational skills learnt, and the video tape produced, are part of the work, but it is the positive change that participants go through during the process that is the most important outcome. This informs the activity and approach at every stage of the work.

Participatory video can have far-reaching benefits. Video utilized in this way can be a potent tool for group empowerment.

> It develops communication within and between groups, and many skills in those taking part. People gain confidence working together, and develop a means of expressing themselves, as well as the belief that they have something worth saying.
>
> (Shaw 1992: 22)

Participatory video is a catalyst for interaction and co-operation, the presence of the camera motivating people to take part. It brings them together by stimulating discussion about issues and ideas. Through expressing themselves on tape, and using the camera to focus on their world, participants' awareness of their situation increases.

As the participants' self-assurance grows, and they form opinions, video provides a means for them to communicate their views to a wider audience. Working co-operatively together to make a tape, group members make decisions, plan and are in charge of their own means of communication. Through this process they develop a recognition of their capacity to achieve results, and this can be the first step towards self-help in other areas.

## The approach

The circumstances of many people's lives have resulted in them having little self-belief and insufficient control over the decisions that affect them. Many were judged failures by an examination-orientated education. Unemployment, homelessness and other inequalities leave people feeling discarded by society. Prejudice towards those with disabilities; racism; break-down in care for those with mental ill-health; isolation by age, by lack of childcare and through sparse rural facilities; the break-up of traditional communities; and marginalization from the consumer world by economic circumstances all take their toll. A large percentage of the population is left feeling impotent – powerless to do things for themselves. Others speak on their behalf and organize things for them. Any approach that seeks to address these people's basic needs must involve engaging with the attitudinal constraints induced in them by this powerlessness. Development work should endeavour to:

- Increase self-esteem and counteract people's tendency to put themselves down.
- Encourage them to try new things and feel proud of their achievements.
- Build confidence in their capacities and ideas, and in their ability to express their opinions, without fear of derision or reproach.
- Encourage trust in the group process, and less deference to those in charge, through a learner-orientated approach.
- Provide problem-solving opportunities to develop their ability to reflect, diagnose, create, decide and act.
- Generate greater self-reliance through the development of decision-making and planning skills.
- Decrease feelings of powerlessness by supporting a transfer of responsibility to the group for the control of their work.
- Develop a sense of identity within the group, and encourage them to work collectively to attain results.
- Provide opportunities for them to represent their views to others, including those in authority.

These objectives are not exclusive to participatory video, since much development work with groups shares the same goals, but the participatory video approach stems from a community arts practice that has a well-defined history in the UK.

## Relationship to community arts

Community arts (now more commonly referred to as participatory arts or arts work with people) grew out of the social, cultural and political activism of the late 1960s. From the very beginning it was defined by its aims and approach, rather than by a specific activity or artform. Participation is essential to the way of working, as it is based on the premise that being actively involved in collective artistic expression can change people's awareness of the world around them, as well as their perception of themselves. 'Art created in a community context can be a transforming influence. This is true especially for those who are disadvantaged or oppressed' (Report of the National Enquiry in the Arts 1992: 29).

Community arts involves 'animateurs' (practitioners, workers, facilitators) working in partnership with a specific community, in a place familiar to the participants. The setting is important. The practitioner works with the group in their own environment (work, domestic or social) rather than requiring them to come to an unfamiliar venue, where they would be less comfortable. An exception may be made where the setting is restrictive and oppressive, and where working somewhere else would be liberating and empowering (page 204). Creative expression is then used as the focus to engage in and communicate the experiences, needs and aspirations of that community. Using both traditional and new artforms, its goals are to stimulate individual development and group identity; to help people explore as yet unrealized capabilities; to contribute to personal, social and environmental change; and to generate self-directed action within the community. It usually takes place in situations of deprivation or disadvantage, where morale may be low, social cohesion lacking and opportunity scarce.

Through the 1970s and early 1980s many community arts practitioners concentrated on working with the communications media, and the community media movement was born. It has been described as

> concerned with building up people's awareness of what is going on around them – constructing a picture of the real world, often with a view to changing it. It is about getting people to help themselves and decide their own futures rather than having their lives controlled for them by external forces.
>
> (Wade 1980: 5)

Print, photography, film, radio and video are very direct ways for marginalized communities to get their message across to a wider audience. Throughout the UK many groups have produced newsletters for their members; posters to advertise events and communicate issues; photographs for leaflets and exhibitions; as well as local papers, radio programmes, films and videos.

The communications media are especially good vehicles for participatory arts work. They combine the benefits of creative expression with a clear channel of communication for the communities concerned, providing an obvious way for them to generate change by voicing their opinions to those with decision-making power.

Video shares its benefits as a development tool with the other communications media. It also has its own specific benefits. Used in a participatory way, it provides an excellent way of amplifying and accelerating some of the group processes involved. Martha Stuart, who worked for many years using video as a tool for social change with women in India, commented on its incredible ability to generate human drive and energy (Stuart 1981: 35).

One of the reasons why video has this potential is because of its relationship with broadcast television. Television is the dominant cultural force in present-day society. It is a primary leisure activity and the prevalent mass medium but, whilst most people watch television, few have any say about its form and content. Production is extremely centralized and controlled by a remote influential elite, providing a predominantly one-way channel of communication.

Video is not the same as television because the control of production is located with the users themselves, but it uses similar technology and can look remarkably alike because it is played back on a television monitor. Participatory video thus links participatory arts practice with this predominant cultural form, and this gives the work added poignancy and power.

## Problems with television

Television is all-pervasive. Everyone knows what it is and the majority have an opinion about it (often divided and strongly felt), but what does it actually do? It must have considerable power, or advertisers would not spend so much money using it to influence buying behaviour, but research into the effects of television watching is fraught with difficulty.

One thing is sure: people spend a considerable proportion of their lives watching television. In 1993 the national weekly average in the UK was 25 hours and 41 minutes (Central Statistical Office 1995: 216). Television must play a major part in reducing participation in other activity as there is simply not much spare time remaining. Beyond this monopolization of time, however, it is not easy to say anything about television viewing with any certainty at all. It is hard to establish exactly how it influences people because its effect seems to depend on the person watching and what they bring to the experience.

Justin Lewis, in *The Ideological Octopus*, has explored past and recent television audience research to assess the progress made in understanding the ideological role television plays in society, and whether it controls us, or we control it.

> At the heart of this debate is a tension between the viewer and the viewed. Where does power – the power to create and solidify meanings – *really* lie? Does it rest in the hands of the TV producer or the TV consumer?
>
> (Lewis 1991: 6)

One of the research difficulties is that it is impossible to isolate any effect as being due solely to television watching, aside from other social factors. In addition, television may change the way people think rather than their behaviour, the effect may be long-term and, importantly, viewers cannot be assumed to receive pre-packaged meanings passively. It is their engagement with television that generates meaning, and different people may derive different meanings from the same programme.

The result of these problems initially shifted the research emphasis to how people use television to satisfy their needs. As Lewis explains, by assuming the viewer has complete control over what they watch, this perspective leads to an inherent contradiction:

> People are, on the one hand, shaped and determined by the social world, instilling them with certain 'values,' 'interests,' 'social roles' and 'associations': and yet, when it comes to watching TV, they appear to suddenly develop the ability to 'select' and 'fashion' what they see and hear in accordance with their interests.
>
> (Lewis 1991: 15–16)

'Cultivation analysis' presented an alternative way round the effects research dilemma. Rather than looking at the effect of television on, for instance, violent behaviour, it looked at the changes in the viewers' perception of violence. This approach managed to produce studies linking television to the cultivation of particular attitudes. For example: 'cultivation analysis has revealed that, in certain countries (notably the US), the more TV you watch, the more likely you are to have a fearful or distrustful attitude to the world outside (Gerbner and Gross, 1976)' (Lewis 1991: 19).

Despite these results, the complexity of the question caused the research focus to shift during the early 1970s to programme content. This resulted in two areas of interest: 'content analysis', which quantitatively assesses how television represents the world; and the more qualitative 'textual analysis', which looks at how the television form creates meanings. Most early textual analysis concentrated on the power of the television message, challenging the presumption that the meaning is self-evident. More recently, cultural studies has brought the audience's background into sharper focus. Defining culture as being expressed in the practices of everyday life, as opposed to the 'high art' view of culture as separate and above the society it relates to, it considers the social and cultural environment in which television watching takes place. Television meanings are now thought to be produced by the active engagement between the television message and the television viewer with reference to their cultural perspective, and recent research has attempted to study the complex relationship between the two.

As awareness of the issues has grown, media researchers have become more and more cautious about making any generalizations about television at all. Further, in the desire to position television as a valid cultural form worthy of serious study, and with the contention that popular genres such as soaps can empower, questioning the medium itself (regardless of the intrinsic value of the content) has become unfashionable, if not taboo.

Even though we do not yet understand television and find it difficult to measure its effects, it is hard to believe that a device that only began life in the first half of the twentieth century, and now plays such a prominent role, cannot but have profound influence. Additionally, the question of the effect of television technology seems to have been lost in the content-based focus of most recent research.

Lewis uses his own studies to suggest that television influences people regardless of whether they understand the message in the way the maker intended, and to contend that just because people derive various messages from a programme does not mean that the audience is in total control. He concludes that: 'To comprehend the power of television . . . we must appreciate its influence regardless of intention and in the face of polysemy [many meanings]' (Lewis 1991: 203).

Jerry Mander goes further. Fifteen years as an advertising executive convinced him of the power of television. His book explores rarely examined aspects of television watching to build up a radical and thought-provoking argument challenging the prevailing view of a benign, neutral instrument to be used or abused.

> I heard many people say, 'Television is great; there are so many things on TV that we'd never otherwise experience.' . . . Yet the television image of the Borneo forest or the news or historical events was surely not the experience of them. . . . It was only the experience of sitting in a darkened room. . . . Because so many of us were confusing television experience with direct experience of the world, we were not noticing that experience itself was being unified to the single behaviour of watching television.
>
> (Mander 1978: 24–6)

Television promotes itself as a window on the world, but it is not a window through which you can touch, smell or feel. Every experience is mediated. Despite the undoubted educational value of some television programmes, and the audience's part in forming meanings, this replacement of direct experience by a unified mediated experience can leave people disconnected from reality. Without knowledge built on first-hand observation, the reliance on television to make sense of the world can increase. People may stop trusting their own experiences, and televised events then gain greater value. Additionally, watching television can isolate people from each other, in the home and in the wider community. Real contact can be replaced by the shared experience of being plugged into the same programmes as others, and as the opportunity for personal interaction decreases, more dependence on the information transmitted is created. By concentrating people on events well outside their lives, which they can do nothing about, television may actually increase feelings of powerlessness.

Television also seems to have a physiological effect. Common experience verifies how difficult it can be to stop viewing once the television is turned on. If you are in a room with it, it is hard to ignore. Your eyes are drawn to it and it is difficult to maintain conversation. Anecdotal reports collated by Mander suggest the experience leaves people feeling drained of energy, mesmerized and hypnotized. He describes how, when watching, pulse and eye movement decreases, the body is stilled, background light and sound are reduced, and communication between watchers is inhibited. He proposes that television in this way locks people to it, dulling the senses and dimming awareness, inducing passivity through the very act of watching (Mander 1978: 158–66).

Through reviewing and following up the available research relating to the physiological effects of television technology, he speculates that the repetitive flickering of the television screen might actually switch off cognitive processing in the left brain cortex, thus inhibiting logical thinking. Bypassing consciousness, television could be pouring a continuous stream of information directly into the head, allowing the right brain to absorb unprocessed images at an emotional level. He argues that this is more akin to brain-washing or sleep-teaching than a critical learning process (Mander 1978: 192–215).

If Mander is correct, television may play a significant part in reducing self-awareness, generating mass inaction and decreasing interaction with others. What is surprising, as Mander highlights, is that whilst uncovering some research to support his ideas and whilst most experts he consulted agreed that, on the basis of their study in related areas, television could have the physiological effects he suggests, he found so little work exploring these questions in depth. Has television so quickly become entrenched in our world that to contemplate that it could be an unhealthy factor in the physical environment, regardless of what it transmits, is heresy?

## THE BENEFITS OF PARTICIPATORY VIDEO

Participatory video uses its connection to television to involve people actively in the world around them. Participatory video can empower because it hands over control of the medium to the participants, using it in a way that subverts the possible effects of television watching. Group members actively do, rather than consume. They see themselves on the screen, and control what happens, rather than observing a distant land. They stop and start the tape rather than being fed with an unending stream of images and information. Isolation from others is broken down through group interaction, and sharing direct experience encourages them to develop their own opinions instead of being told what to think. In essence, participatory video aims to transform the feelings of powerlessness that may have been fostered and stimulates participants to take more control over their lives.

To explore video's potential benefits as a development tool, participatory video practice can be divided into eight major elements:

- Participation
- Individual development
- Communication
- Community building
- Critical awareness and consciousness raising
- Self-advocacy and representation
- Capacity development and self-reliance
- Empowerment

Before examining these benefits in more detail it is worth emphasizing the basis on which they are presented. Although the approaches and techniques described in this book have been developing since the 1970s, participatory video is still a relatively new discipline. As with much group work, the practice is in advance of more rigorous validation. The analysis is not therefore intended to be rigidly definitive. The practice theory developed has been found to be empirically effective, and provides a broad-based hypothetical framework that can inform further work and the assessment of future experience.

## Participation

> this process must subordinate media to people's decisions and needs. The media production techniques, the information that comes through the media, the achievement of a final video or other media, must be secondary aims subordinated to the process whereby people have a real opportunity to develop themselves.
>
> (Corrêa da Silva 1988: 69)

Participation implies an active engagement in the world: doing rather than observing. It involves joining with others to make decisions, to set objectives and to plan and take local action.

Stimulating participation is a primary goal of development work. The fragmented contemporary western lifestyle has resulted in many people lacking a sense of belonging both to their local community and to the wider society. They are displaced from their roots, isolated from their neighbours and disillusioned with the political processes that affect them. Worldwide, many people have little control over their destinies because their lives are dictated by outside social and economic circumstances.

Involving disadvantaged people is often the hardest part of any development process, precisely because of the apathy and lack of inertia generated by their powerlessness. If they have no sense of identification or involvement, they may doubt that the work is directed at them, or feel it holds no relevance. If they have low self-regard they may believe that they have nothing to offer, or fear failure. In other words, the reasons why people do not take part can be the very reasons that work with them is needed.

In order to generate meaningful participation, development work cannot simply be imposed from above on passive recipients. It is crucial that people take an active part in decisions affecting their development. When 'outside' workers intervene, participants must understand the purpose of the work and the role they will play in it. A mechanism should be set up that allows them to define their needs and responds to their input so that they are involved in controlling the direction of the work.

Video can be particularly good at encouraging active involvement. It is a form of creative expression accessible to all, regardless of literacy, creative confidence or academic achievement. The approach is non-exclusive, learner-orientated and enabling. Even those who are initially hesitant soon find they can succeed.

Applied with a participatory approach, video can be highly motivating. The themes explored through the process are grounded in the participants' lives. This places them at the very centre of the action, because it revolves around their experiences and needs, and consequently generates its own sense of purpose.

Participatory video thus provides a means for participants to define the issues that are important to them, which can give them ownership of the work right from the start. It then aims systematically to hand over control of the process to the group, providing structure without imposing content. Their opinions and decision-making skills are developed in a way that gives them real choices with full comprehension of the opportunities available to them.

These factors make video an extremely good tool for participation. It can be used to stimulate the development process, bringing the group together and motivating them to participate further.


## Individual development

people . . . use their newly found confidence, and awareness of themselves and their surroundings, in a greater ability to make decisions in other areas of their lives.

(Shaw 1986: 7)

Participatory video aims to facilitate individual growth through the context of the group process. The approach stimulates self-expression from the beginning. Everybody is given the opportunity to speak, and because participants are asked to talk about themselves, they all have things to say.

Recording their experiences and ideas on tape assists a process of self-definition. Video acts as a mirror. Playing back the recorded material can promote reflection and develop a sense of self.

Videoing someone can be a valuing process in itself. A focused camera picks them out from the crowd, recognizing them as an individual. All participants contribute to the video material recorded and everyone's piece is equally valued. This boosts confidence that they have something worth saying, and helps them develop thoughts and form opinions. The positive feedback they receive increases their self-esteem and they become more able to express their ideas fluently.

Video production provides the opportunity to acquire many technical, creative and social skills. The fact that participants are provided with the chance to succeed at new challenges is more important, however, than the learning of a particular skill. Using video can be particularly confidence-building. Many people think they will not be able to use the equipment or speak on tape but immediate playback generates almost instant results. Getting feedback straight-away enables participants to learn very quickly, improving on their technique, and further building confidence in their capabilities. Encouraging participants to recognize their achievements can develop an awareness of their potential.

## Communication

> Video also makes possible the opening of a sideward flow of communication – the channel of people talking with each other. Video facilitates exchange within communities, between communities. And beyond this, it allows people to talk back and up the ladder of communication – to leaders, to policy-makers.
>
> (Atienza 1977: 12)

Communication can be a one-way process, with information passing predominantly in one direction. In this case the communicator intends to affect the audience by expressing their message. One-way communication can be face-to-face, as with a speech or lecture, or via a communication medium such as print, radio or television.

Alternatively, communication can be a two-way process with information passed backwards and forwards, as in conversation and discussion. Two-way communication is a vital component of human activity. Through dialogue people exchange information, ideas, experiences and feelings, and make sense of the world around them.

Participatory development must involve communication between the participants. They discover their own views through considering together issues of concern rather than being told what to think.

Video can stimulate two-way communication. The presence of the equipment generates discussion by giving a reason for talking about issues. Exercises encourage participants to interact with each other very directly by asking questions and making statements. Speaking, interviewing and other communication skills are developed through this process.

Most group work involves discussion but using video can formalize this process, giving it extra weight and meaning. Participants explore topics that they would not usually consider, and concentrate on developing ideas. The formality also ensures that all the participants have an input. The work is structured so that some people do not dominate the discussion whilst others always remain quiet, because each person has the opportunity to speak on the microphone. Everyone expresses opinions and asks questions, and participants are prevented from all talking at once. This can create equal access to the communication process for the entire group.

Participatory video can also be used to develop participants' beliefs. Discussions, opinion statements and interviews are recorded. In this way video acts as a sketch pad, storing every contribution for future reference. Feedback and further thought can be generated by playback, and used to take a discussion forward by exploring attitudes expressed, or following up particular themes.

Video can stimulate communication between people who would not otherwise interact. Participants can use it to talk to those outside the group, as well as to each other. As a visual and spoken medium, it can be used by illiterate people and to develop non-verbal communication.

Communication does not have to be face-to-face. Video can provide links in the community, through the exchange of recorded tapes. It can increase communication between the participants and those in authority. It thus facilitates debate, consultation and the flow of information.

## Community building

> In sharing there is strength. By exchanging perspectives and experiences, [people] validate reality and the importance of a particular commonality binding them together. . . .
>
> (Stuart 1981: 35)

Group development is a primary goal of participatory video work. The purpose is to promote trust, understanding, co-operation and group cohesion.

During a video project group members talk, listen and exchange perspectives.

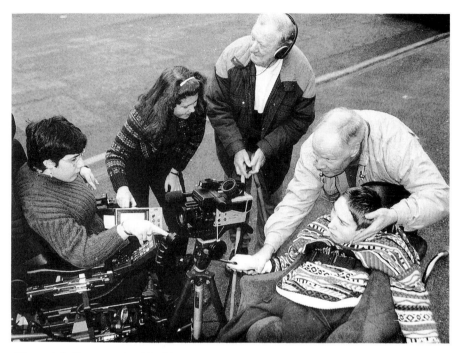

*Figure 1.1* Group work with video

Exploring shared experiences, and establishing common ground, helps to develop a coherent group identity. Participants acquire a feeling of belonging through their shared interests, and a strength from the common bond.

Working together in a supportive environment promotes further trust in the group process. From this position of safety, with a base in common concerns and goals, group members can also investigate areas of difference. This can lead to mutual understanding between them, a tolerance of difference, and greater social cohesion.

Working with video equipment can in itself encourage co-operation. Video is a team activity. Participants have to work co-operatively together to attain a worthwhile result, involving joint planning and decision making. Producing a video programme as a group makes it apparent what working with others can accomplish. This can build new communities, as well as reinvigorating old ones.

## Critical awareness and consciousness raising

> [video] can undoubtedly be a very significant consciousness-raising process for disadvantaged people.
>
> (Shaw 1986: 7)

Video is good at focusing attention because it concentrates participants on what they are seeing and hearing. One image, piece of sound or question is considered at a time, magnifying its impact.

Additionally, video can stimulate interaction between the group and their surroundings. They go out with the equipment, and choose and record shots depending on their perception of what is present.

Exploration with the video equipment encourages participants to examine the world around them, raising their awareness of their position within it. Through this process they start to ask questions and this can lead, in a safe and often humorous way, to critical enquiry into the conditions of their lives.

Agreeing on a topic for a video or a message to convey can increase a group's understanding of what it thinks about an issue. Identifying problems together is often the first stage in making changes. The shared strength can motivate people to continue working together to bring about improvements.

## Self-advocacy and representation

> an element of fairness and justice is brought to communications and the voiceless will start to be heard
>
> (Hénaut 1975: 8)

The majority of people do not have access to a means of voicing their opinions more widely, particularly to those in authority. By giving participants the opportunity to speak up for themselves, video can develop self-advocacy.

As a project progresses, the group's desire to say something to a wider audience often increases. Video used as an organized and disciplined form of investigation helps the construction and ordering of ideas. Participatory video not only raises awareness, it can also enable the group to take action by providing the means for them to represent their viewpoint to a chosen audience and to produce a tape about their concerns.

It is not necessary to spend months making a video programme. This book describes techniques that enable simple but effective communications to be produced in a relatively short time. Group members can develop full control over their work based on a practical understanding of the medium. As the project progresses, they are encouraged to think about the audience, the style of the

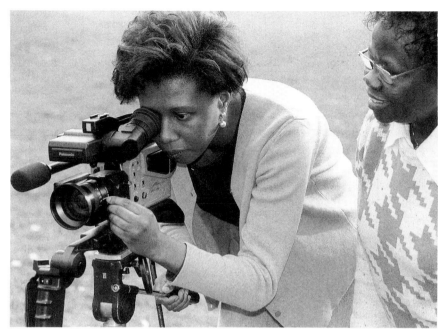

*Figure 1.2* Videoing on location

programme, and the language used, heightening their ability to represent themselves effectively.

## Capacity development and self-reliance

> Video is especially useful when people have a feeling of hopelessness, who don't talk much because they see no hope of change. Once they start talking about their problems they see they are not alone with them, which is the first step to finding solutions.
>
> (Hénaut 1971: 21)

The opportunity to take responsibility is limited for many people, especially those in institutionalized settings. This can make them doubt their own abilities. Recent reorganization in society means that decisions are being thrust on people who have had little preparation for the changes. It is no wonder that many feel bewildered by the new choices facing them.

A primary goal of participatory video work is to develop participants' self-determination, and give them skills to take responsibility for the decisions affecting them.

Working with video generates problem-solving opportunities on a technical, creative, organizational and social level. The exercises used develop the participants' capacity to initiate, diagnose, contemplate, evaluate and take action. Thinking can be clarified, and decision-making and planning skills cultivated.

Using the equipment can give a means to confront the world and enable participants to move in a questioning way in and out of their institutions or everyday environments. They are in charge of technical equipment, with significant production jobs to execute. Roles normally assumed by others can be taken on, and responsibilities exchanged.

From the very beginning of a project, the group are all required to make decisions, and as their planning skills grow, there is a shifting of responsibility for the direction of the project from the workers to the group members. This process can generate a greater self-reliance, stimulating participants to act independently. Formulating and implementing goals can empower participants to make changes in their lives and plan for the future.

## Empowerment

> Small format video ... especially when combined with social animation, holds enormous potential for allowing people to articulate their needs, see themselves, build up their confidence and, finally, work together on solving their problems.
>
> (McLellan 1987: 144)

Empowerment implies that people not only have the capacity to make changes but that they actually do act to influence society and transform their situation.

All the other benefits of video can be seen to contribute towards empowerment. By stimulating the seven responses we have considered above (participation; individual development; communication; community building; critical awareness and consciousness raising; self-advocacy and representation; and capacity development and self-reliance) participatory video can prepare participants to take action.

By developing the work further, the group can progress with increased strength and power to use video as a means to participate in decisions affecting their lives, to communicate with and influence the prevailing power structures, and to bring about changes on an organizational, environmental or political level.

# Participatory video checklist

In essence, participatory video:

- Is a tool for development work.
- Is active rather than passive.
- Is group-based, promoting co-operative working.
- Is grounded in participants' experience and revolves around their needs and ideas.
- Stimulates creative expression.
- Develops confidence and self-esteem.
- Generates interaction and discussion.
- Builds group identity and cohesion.
- Increases awareness and critical enquiry.
- Provides a means to communicate with others.
- Cultivates participants' capabilities and potential.
- Develops planning and decision-making skills.
- Transfers control and responsibility to participants.
- Encourages self-determination of goals.
- Facilitates empowerment.

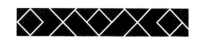

# Workshops

Video offers many benefits when used as a participatory tool for group development work. So what is actually done with the equipment to achieve this potential?

At this point it must be noted that using the medium does not automatically bring success. Video is only a tool, not a process in itself. It cannot do development work, or magically deliver a desired result. To be of value it must be employed by a group worker in an appropriate way.

Some video work with groups is participatory and some is not. In fact, precisely because video is such a powerful medium it is open to abuse, and it can be used very badly. Often this is for the simple reason that workers are unaware of the effect that video has on people and of the possible pitfalls.

This section of the book aims to maximize the value of participatory video work by explaining exactly what to do with the equipment in a group situation, including the mistakes to avoid. It looks practically at the steps involved in facilitating an effective video workshop, covering the general approach, as well as instructions for games and exercises to use at each stage of the process.

# Chapter 2

# Basics

This chapter details basic participatory video practice, providing a practical framework to use throughout, and laying a solid foundation for the work.

It describes the ground rules to establish with the group, the equipment set-up for a standard workshop, and the essential technical and organizational procedure for a video exercise.

## GENERAL APPROACH

The aim is to set up participatory working conditions in which individual growth and group development can flourish.

### The workshop situation

A workshop is a group-based environment in which participants are actively engaged in experiential learning. A task-orientated approach creates opportunities for the group members to develop their latent abilities.

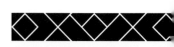

enjoyment of the learning process is an essential condition for its success. To be enjoyable, the learning experiences have to be relevant, purposeful, vital, interactive, challenging, exciting, evocative, and preferably multisensory, hands-on; in short, capable of engaging the learners in every possible way.

(Srinivasan 1992: 50)

Workshops should be pleasurable, stimulating and inspiring, providing the opportunity for participants to succeed at new skills. The atmosphere should be supportive and enabling, maximizing participation and creating equality of access for all group members. The sessions should be lively and light-hearted, based in the participants' experience, and responding to their interests.

In this respect video workshops are the same as other group-based participatory sessions. Video is, however, a very specific, and relatively complicated tool, which adds an extra aspect to the dynamic. It is particularly important to consider how to integrate it, so that it augments rather than negates the participatory process. In particular, a video workshop should:

- *Create an encouraging and reassuring atmosphere* Initially people can feel unconfident both in front of and behind the camera, and all too self-critical. Feedback should be positive. Tell participants what they have done well, rather than concentrating on mistakes (page 231).
- *Introduce technical skills in an accessible way* The approach should be non-academic, non-jargonistic, and provide as much hands-on experience as possible (pages 232–5).
- *Create equal opportunity for all the participants* Some group members can be reluctant to take on certain roles. They may attempt to take refuge behind the camera so that they do not appear on tape, or they may try to avoid using the equipment. Ensure that everyone has equal access to all the roles.
- *Encourage co-operation* Video used badly can bring out competitiveness and lack of respect for others. Production is essentially a team activity so set up co-operative working practices. Encourage mutual support by making sure that participants listen to each other, and intervene if they start undermining one another.

## A structured approach

Above all else, a participatory video session needs to be structured. In all probability participants will not have any idea what video involves and what is possible. If there is no structure, the chances are that the group will try one or two things; then, after the initial excitement of seeing themselves on video, they will become bored and disillusioned. If unstructured work continues, either the activity becomes chaotic and meaningless, or nothing at all gets done. Both alternatives are unproductive, so there is no sense of achievement and motivation quickly evaporates.

Most groups find unstructured work a disempowering experience. It is a misconception that handing the equipment over to participants like this gives them any real control over their work. They must be provided with the necessary skills and some experience of the range of options, for choices to be meaningful.

Operating within a structure means that the workers can make sure that video is used positively rather than in a more objectifying way. The framework ensures that everyone has the same chances to use the equipment, to appear on camera, to voice their opinion, to be heard, to take part in the decision-making process, and that work takes place co-operatively.

Problem-solving tasks can be set up through which group members develop their abilities and try out new skills. Each exercise stretches them further, yet challenges them appropriately so that they succeed. Organized activities produce products on tape very quickly, teaching the members a great deal in a short space of time, and immediately generating a feeling of accomplishment.

A structured approach leads the group through the video process in a way that gradually gives them more control over the work, based on a practical understanding of the options. Organization does not take away responsibility, or stop ideas developing. Instead it supplies a framework to guarantee that participants do expand their creativity, and facilitates a progressive transfer of control to the group as a whole, not just one or two members.

The structure also responds to the group's motivations. The organizational and technical procedures are dictated by the exercises, but the content is supplied by the experiences, ideas and interests of the group.

## Workers' attitude

Running a participatory video workshop requires a range of skills and experience. Workers must be able to:

- Facilitate participatory group work.
- Be supportive and encouraging.
- Develop communication skills.
- Plan activities yet be adaptable and responsive to the situation.
- Use video equipment flexibly, and produce programmes co-operatively.
- Teach hands-on technical skills (see Chapter 9).
- Provide strong leadership yet gradually transfer responsibility to the group.

One of the biggest factors contributing to the success of a video project is the attitude that the workers have to the people in the group. Indeed, two workers with different perspectives can run the same exercise with opposite effects.

> The attitudes that a worker with people has towards them contributes substantially to their development or lack of development. People respond to their perception of attitudes as these are expressed in gesture, word, and deed.... The beliefs he [the worker] holds about human beings and his intentions, stated or implied, are important to the outcome in people's lives.
>
> (Biddle and Biddle 1966: 58)

If the workers have low expectations of the participants' capabilities, low attainment is almost inevitable. If the workers have high expectations, and expect them to do well, then they are more likely to fulfil their potential.

The participatory group development process is based on an optimistic attitude towards people. Each individual is seen as having unique possibilities, valuable undeveloped abilities, and the capacity to grow and develop through the process. Biddle and Biddle suggest that the worker's belief in people has to be genuinely felt, reflecting their underlying philosophy, and compare their belief to the rapport needed for a successful therapeutic relationship (Biddle and Biddle 1966: 59).

The outcome of a project is thus affected by any pre-conceived expectations. Avoiding assumptions is especially important with video work as its technical nature leads to stereotypical notions about who is able to do it. Individuals commonly accomplish things in a video session that staff members thought they were incapable of doing.

As a worker you should endeavour to be as impartial as possible and to keep an open mind. Avoid making judgements about groups and individuals based on stereotypes, other workers' comments, or your own experience of similar groups. While it can be necessary to get background information about a group before working with them, knowledge about their previous accomplishments should not affect your working practice.

Workers or staff who know a group well inevitably have opinions about them. It is then more difficult not to anticipate outcomes. This is also true for a worker who is familiar with a particular type of client group. Remember that groups sharing certain characteristics are not identical, and that the same group can react differently to a new experience. Try to provide opportunities for all group members to succeed.

## PARTICIPATORY VIDEO PRACTICE

The practice theory contained in this book is a practical methodology that has been found to be effective in achieving the aims of participatory video work with groups. This does not mean that there is only one correct way of working. Nonetheless the techniques are suggested because they have proved to be of value during face-to-face work, and are not just the result of abstract theorizing. The working practice that follows has shown itself useful with a wide variety of groups, in many diverse situations.

In order for participants to take part constructively, the boundaries within which they are operating need to be apparent. In an unfamiliar setting some clear ground rules based on the working methodology give them an understanding of what is expected of them in the workshop. Maintaining a consistent approach helps to ensure that the sessions are a success.

The following simple rules provide an extremely solid and effective basis for participatory video work. Adhering to them from the very beginning avoids a lot of the problems that might otherwise occur. It is not usually necessary to recite them to the group; instead they should be implicit in the way the work is organized and carried out. Most essentially there must be consistency in their application. Ground rules should be over-ridden only in exceptional circumstances and with the full support of the group.

The ground rules below apply to the use of video. There may be others relating to acceptable workshop behaviour that you will want to agree with the group.

## Ground rules

### *Participants always operate the equipment themselves*

A fundamental aim of the work is to hand over skills to the group so that they are in control of their own communications. Group members learn technical skills through practical experience (page 232), so it is vital that they use the equipment themselves from the very start. If the workers use the equipment, and video the group, the project is not participatory.

Do not begin by giving a lecture explaining how to use video. All this achieves is to alienate participants further from the equipment and discourage them from trying. Instead set up activities that give everyone direct experience of handling and operating the equipment as soon as possible. Use games and exercises to provide the maximum opportunity for them all to gain confidence of videoing in an unpressurized way.

## Everyone attending must agree to appearing on video

Participants, workers, and anyone else present at the workshop, must be willing to be videoed and see themselves on screen. This is fundamental to a participatory use of video. If you are going to video other people, you must be prepared to be recorded yourself. It is iniquitous to put others through something that you are disinclined to face.

Of course most people feel embarrassed when they first watch themselves on tape. If one or two people bravely volunteer to appear alone, nobody else gets used to the feeling; and if anyone avoids appearing once, it is doubly difficult to persuade them to participate in the future.

Before the project starts, make everybody aware that it involves being videoed. If anyone refuses to appear during the session, make it quite clear that it is a condition of entry to the group. If they continue to resist, ask them to leave, and stop until they go. (You are unlikely to discourage those who genuinely want to join the project as long as it is obvious that you are serious.)

It is essential that workshop leaders and any other staff attending appear on camera alongside everybody else. You must show a willingness to put yourself through the same experiences as the group, and share any feelings of embarrassment.

Clearly, any spectators will undermine the trust that is being created amongst group members. Funders and managers who want to see how the work is going must also join in. Evaluation should be built into the project (page 208), and it may be necessary to point out that it is inappropriate for outsiders to come into sessions early in the project, as it interferes with the group's development at a crucial stage. (They can come back later on when the group is more settled, and then it can provide a useful opportunity for participants to present their work.)

If anyone else comes into the room during the session and tries to watch, stop and wait until they leave. (They normally go quite quickly when there is nothing to see except everyone staring at them.) If it is impossible to continue without spectators, you will have to reassess the viability of the project setting.

## Participants take turns at every role

All the roles in front of and behind the camera are rotated to ensure that all the participants have the opportunity to learn every skill.

Some workers suggest that each individual should stick to one role to become really proficient at it. In practice this means that only the most confident participants become skilled at the favoured roles. Everyone must have an equal chance to develop, so swapping around is essential.

Most groups have one or two members who want to do everything first.

Taking turns prevents these individuals from dominating the workshop by monopolizing the camera or the workers' time. Make it clear that everyone gets a go at everything so there is no need to push.

Swapping also creates space for the more reticent members to participate fully, and can generate a co-operative rather than a competitive environment. For example, on a video project at one summer playscheme a boy repeatedly tried to push others off the equipment. Once he realized that he was not going to be allowed another go until everyone else had had their turn, he became a positive asset. Not only did he remember who had used the camera, and in what order, but he also actively encouraged the less confident members to take part. He could have destroyed the workshop if the ground rules had not been firmly established from the start, but instead his energy and enthusiasm were channelled constructively.

Most people consider the camera operator to be the most important and powerful position. This is especially true when using a camcorder (page 237). Consequently, it is essential that all the participants have a go on the camera during each session, and that they have the same number of turns overall. Even if an individual is particularly unconfident, and says that they do not want to use the equipment, insist that they do. It may seem easier to wait until next time, but unless you overcome the resistance immediately, their fear will simply increase, and it is then even harder to get them on the camera subsequently. Offer to help by operating the camera with them, and they are unlikely to refuse.

There may be occasions when it is difficult for the whole group to operate the camera in a single session (e.g. if the group is very large or time is short). Make it plain that those remaining will be first next session, and stick to your word.

## Play back everything recorded in its entirety

You may be tempted to speed up the play-back process by skipping forward through workshop material, especially if the game went on too long or did not work as well as usual, or if you have watched an exercise many times before with other groups. Remember that seeing themselves is a new and fascinating experience for those participating. At the start of a project the group members have a voracious appetite for watching themselves. This is an important part of the development process, and playing back everything recorded in full is crucial.

If you fast-forward through any of the tape, it sends a strong negative message to the group. It implies that their work is not worth watching. The individuals who appear in the missed material can feel that they are of no interest, and those operating the equipment can think that their efforts were inadequate. Confidence is destroyed when the goal is to build it up.

Take viewing time into account when planning the workshop, and as a rule do not start an exercise unless there is time to watch the recording.

## Never video other people without permission

The group must always ask permission if they want to video other people. Uphold this as the only acceptable way of working, and do not allow the equipment to be used otherwise. This ground rule is central to ethical video production work. Empowering the group so that they abuse their position in the way they treat other people is not the goal. If necessary, discuss how they might feel if videoed without consent, and explain how treating their subject with respect produces better results.

When permission is sought, the person concerned should be given a distinct choice, with no coercion, however well meaning. Describe the purpose of the recording, and how it is going to be used. If it is part of a workshop exercise, it can help to explain the project goals. If the finished video is going to be shown more widely, ask if they are happy for it to be edited; written permission is also strongly advised.

In fact, the participatory video approach generally involves the group making videos about themselves. They are both producer and subject. This is very different from traditional video production where the programme makers control the process from behind the camera, and 'take' pictures of their 'subject', often unaware of, or exploiting, their position of power. Using the participatory approach makes the participants more supportive even when they video people outside the group.

## Video material recorded in the workshop is confidential

Any workshop material recorded on tape is part of a development process. As such it should be treated as confidential. For the group to participate fully they must be able to trust that no one else is going to watch the tape produced without their permission.

Later on in the project the participants may want to show their work to people outside the group. Make sure that this is with everyone's full knowledge and consent, and that the presentation is under their control.

## Preparation

### *Project planning*

A participatory video project requires careful planning. In fact its success rests heavily on thorough preparation. Before the sessions begin, the following components should be considered and organized:

- Aims and goals of the project
- Group membership
- Workers
- Project structure
- Venue
- Equipment and other resources
- Management, administration and funding
- Evaluation and monitoring

These factors are explored in depth in Chapter 7.


### *Project workers*

At this point it is worth considering the number of workers needed to run a participatory video project effectively.

Most group work benefits from having two workers because there are two distinct types of facilitative role: that of task leader co-ordinates the specific group activity and that of emotional leader develops and maintains the way in which participants work together by cultivating communication, co-operation, trust and group relationships (Douglas 1976: 70–1). These roles are not necessarily mutually exclusive, and can be combined in one worker, but there are lots of advantages in having co-leaders. Two different perspectives can assist planning, problem solving and evaluation. Within the session both workers can fulfil independent functions at the same time; both can support the other's interaction with the group; both can take over if the other is in difficulty; and one can deal with individuals on a one-to-one basis whilst the other carries on with the rest of the group.

Two workers are even more desirable when running participatory video projects because there are essentially two distinct functions for workers to perform in addition to the facilitative roles. One involves teaching technical skills to the participants, and supporting their use of the equipment; the other entails organizing the activity in front of the camera. To keep the group actively involved these functions need to take place simultaneously.

Video can be quite slow for those who are not using the equipment. If only one worker is available, it is very difficult to keep the whole group engaged and busy at all times. While the lone worker shows the camera operator how to use the camera, the rest of the group is unoccupied. They are likely to lose motivation quite quickly. Meanwhile the camera operator is under considerable pressure because everyone else is watching them prepare. The worker then has to help the sound recordist and other equipment operators get ready, and finally to organize the activity in front of the camera. It is easy to see how the group can spend much of the session sitting around waiting.

In addition, a hands-on video session is multilayered, intense and demanding. The process requires considerable interactivity, responsiveness and flexibility on the part of the workers. One facilitator simply has too many things to do, and can easily feel overwhelmed. Two workers are consequently strongly recommended, even with small groups. With two workers everyone is kept active for the majority of the time, the pace is kept up, and the session is involving and interesting, inspiring participants to continue.

There can be considerable financial pressure to use a single worker, but remember that a half-hour workshop with two workers is a far more satisfying and constructive experience than a one-hour session with one worker.

If there is only one worker available with participatory video skills, a co-worker may be able to support the group work. Find out if a member of staff at the project setting is available to assist in this way. Alternatively, particularly if the group is more established, a natural leader within the group may be able to take some responsibility for the process.

## Workshop planning

Each workshop session is part of the overall project plan developed from the project aims. The project plan is developed according to the length and frequency of the sessions, the duration of the project, the nature of the group and the process they are to go through to meet the goals of the project. Chapter 8 outlines the factors to consider when producing the project plan.

## Before the session

Thorough consultation should already have taken place to iron out any difficulties before the project starts (Chapter 7). Ensure that the participants are given all the information and support that they need prior to the first session. Everyone should understand enough about the project to know what to expect. Having said this, too much talking can build apprehension. A taster session is the best way for people to find out what is involved in video (page 196), and decide if they want to take part in the project.

To make sure all the arrangements are clear, contact the group again one or two days before the session. Reconfirm the suitability and availability of the venue, and any travel or childcare provisions. Most important of all, check the equipment well before the session. You need to be competent and confident in its use. If it is unfamiliar, allocate additional time to practise (pages 231–2).

On the day, arrive in time to arrange the room and set up the equipment. Check it is working yourself before the workshop starts. Do not rely on someone else. Video equipment is notoriously badly looked after, and can arrive with vital bits missing. Make sure you have enough time to deal with any problems before the group arrives.

## Standard equipment set-up and workshop lay-out

When the group first meets it is a good idea to have the equipment set up and ready to go so that they can start using it straight away. In all the later sessions it is important that the participants help carry the equipment in and get it ready. Either way the equipment and the chairs should be laid out as shown in Figure 2.1. If there are windows in the room, position the equipment in front of and facing away from them, so that the light falls on the group. Ensure that there are no windows or bright lights behind the group, which would cause backlighting problems during the workshop (page 258).

Place the camera on a tripod set at a height of about 1 metre (3ft 3in), convenient for use by a person sitting down. The camera is then at eye level for the seated group. This is the most appropriate angle for the initial exercises (page 264); the camera operator does not tower over the group; and wheelchair users or people who have difficulty standing are not discriminated against when they use the camera.

Most video viewfinders are on the left of the camera body. The camera operator generally uses their right hand to hold the tripod arm and their left to zoom and focus (page 247). The monitor (page 237) and other equipment is placed on a table to the right of the camera body (the opposite side to the viewfinder). This means that the worker can show the operator how to use the camera, whilst both the operator and the worker can see the monitor.

Make sure that the tripod is close to the table so that participants cannot walk between the camera and the table and trip over any leads between them. The table and the tripod provide a secure base for the equipment, so that it is less likely to get damaged, and the group can easily access the equipment functions.

Position the chairs in a semi-circle, equidistant from the camera. This places all the seated participants at the same distance from the lens, and thus at the same

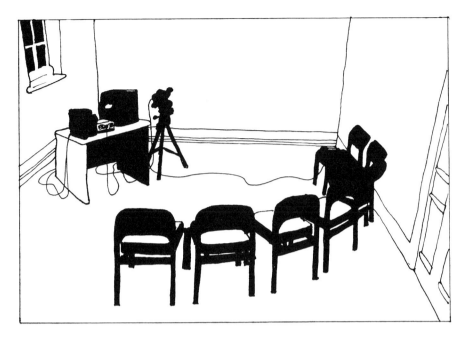

*Figure 2.1* Standard workshop lay-out

focal distance. If the camera operator focuses on one person, everyone else will be in focus as well (pages 247–9).

Make sure that there are enough chairs for all the participants and the workers. Leave adequate space and manoeuvring room for wheelchair users around the chairs and the equipment.

Place the monitor so that the camera operator can see the screen (see Figure 2.2), but those in front of the camera cannot. It is very off-putting and distracting if those in front of the camera are able to see themselves on the monitor while being videoed. Turn the monitor around to play back tapes, and afterwards turn it back again for the next camera operator.

Turn the sound on the monitor up for playback, but completely down during recording, otherwise the sound from the microphone feeds back through the monitor speakers, creating an excruciating noise.

Wire up the equipment (page 241). Make sure that the hand-mike lead is long enough to reach the participants when they are seated on the chairs.

Make sure that all cabling and leads are safely out of the way so that participants cannot trip over them when they move around during the workshop. If possible, given the lighting conditions and the room shape, set up the equipment near to the power sockets, so that long extension leads are not needed. Run cables along walls rather than across the middle of the floor, and try not to

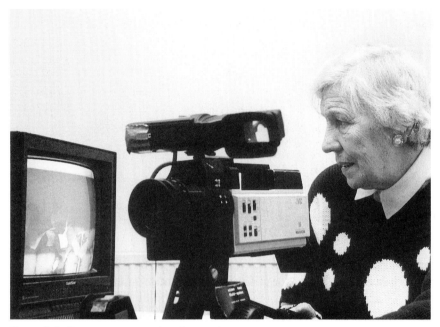

*Figure 2.2* Camera operator using the monitor

run them in front of doors, emergency exits or where the group is likely to walk. Where this is unavoidable, use strong adhesive tape (gaffer tape) to stick leads to the floor.

Power up the equipment, white balance, and do a test recording to make sure that everything is working before the group arrives (Chapter 9).

This standard equipment set-up and room lay-out is used for all exercises and games unless otherwise specified. Early workshops always start and finish with this format to bring the group together at the beginning and end of a session. This only changes much later on in a project, when the group is in the middle of production work and goes straight out. Then it is still useful to use the set-up to round off the session with a final exercise, or to watch what has been recorded.

## Standard exercise procedure

The main activity in a participatory video project consists of a number of video exercises. Games and exercises are used to teach basic equipment techniques, to develop ideas and communication skills, to encourage co-operation and responsibility within the group, and to achieve individual and group development.

Video games and exercises throughout the participatory process follow a standard pattern unless otherwise specified. The customary procedure is as follows.

Two workers facilitate the exercise. One (the activity leader) organizes the action in front of the camera, whilst the other (the technical worker) works with the camera operator to show them how to use the camera. The whole group is occupied, and an intimate one-to-one space is created around the camera. The camera operator can concentrate on using the camera without feeling under pressure, and the rest of the group do not get bored waiting.

Ideally, the two workers swap technical and activity organizing roles through the session, so that they both take part fully in all elements of the process.

At the start, the technical worker for that exercise finds a camera operator by asking, 'Who wants to use the camera first/next?' During the early stages of the project, when all the participants are learning about the equipment, show the camera operator how to pan and tilt the camera with the tripod, how to focus (make the picture clear), how to move the zoom lever to frame the shot, and how to switch the camera on and off (pages 271–5). Then set the equipment in record mode before the start of the exercise (page 252).

Later on in the process, get the camera operator to set the equipment in record mode themselves; support them on the camera, reminding them of any camera procedures they have forgotten; and teach any additional skills according to the exercise.

The activity leader explains the exercise to the rest of the group, organizes the action, and helps participants prepare. Any further equipment roles are supported by either worker, depending on who is available at the time.

When preparation is complete, the exercise begins. The camera operator starts the camera on a pre-arranged signal, and the activity is recorded. The activity leader takes part fully in front of the camera. The technical worker joins in nearer the end of the game if the camera operator seems confident enough to finish the recording without direct support.

At the end, the camera operator switches the camera off (page 253) and then rewinds the recorded exercise to the beginning (page 253), while the other worker makes sure that those in front of the camera are seated in a position where they can see and hear the monitor.

The monitor is turned round, the sound turned up, and the recording played back. Finally, feedback and discussion take place. The workers raise points as appropriate depending on the material recorded and how the participants respond.

If there is to be another exercise, change camera operator, and any other technical and production roles; turn the monitor back again, and the sound down; set up the equipment in record mode; and repeat the procedure.

# Basics checklist

*General approach*

- Make workshops enjoyable, exciting and motivating.
- Create a supportive and enabling atmosphere.
- Take a positive attitude and build confidence.
- Encourage co-operation and develop mutual trust.
- Provide equality of access for all participants.
- Structure work to generate success at new tasks.
- Pass on technical skills through active experience.
- Do not limit achievement by attitude or expectation.

*Ground rules*

- Participants always operate the equipment themselves.
- Everyone at the session appears on video.
- Participants take turns at all roles.
- All video recorded is played back.
- Other people must not be videoed without permission.
- Video recorded in the session is confidential.

*Workshops*

- Be clear about the aims of projects and workshops.
- Ensure thorough planning of video sessions.
- Use two workers.
- Decide in advance who is responsible for what.
- Be flexible and responsive to the group.
- Ensure equipment is working before the session.

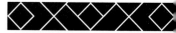

*Equipment set-up and general procedure*

- Lay out the equipment and room appropriately.
- Initially set up equipment ready for the group. In all the later sessions get the group to carry it in and set it up themselves.
- White balance and do a test recording before starting the session.
- One worker teaches the person using the camera. The other organizes the activity.
- Turn the monitor away from those in front of the camera during recording, and back again to view.
- Turn the monitor sound down for recording to avoid feedback.
- Always play everything back immediately.
- Swap technical roles every exercise.

# Initial contact

This chapter looks at the early practical activity in a participatory video project. First it examines the familiarization stage of the process, exploring the important factors to consider during the initial contact with the group. Afterwards it suggests a series of introductory games to use at the first session, and explains why they are recommended.

Next it describes how these fundamental game structures provide an organizational and technical framework for the work, showing how they can be adapted and reutilized throughout the project. Lastly it outlines how self-expression is developed by the early games.

## FAMILIARIZATION

Familiarization is the first stage of the participatory video process. It lays the groundwork for the whole project. During this phase of development participants become familiar with the workshop situation and what is expected of them. They get to know each other and the workers, acquiring trust in the group process, and

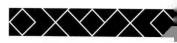

they gain initial experience using the equipment and seeing themselves on video.

It is important not to rush this early work. It is quite usual for people to feel initially inhibited in a workshop environment, especially if it is a new experience, or they do not know each other. The addition of video equipment greatly exaggerates these feelings. The participants need time and space to overcome any discomfort generated by the camera's presence.

The familiarization games and exercises act as ice-breakers, relieving any tension and generating a relaxed mood. Everyone watches themselves on video, possibly for the first time, which is a significant moment.

In addition, familiarization sets the scene for the entire project by establishing the general approach and the ground rules. It introduces standard equipment operations, organizational procedures and working methods, providing a strong foundation for the work.

## Familiarization practice

As long as it is approached sensitively, video work is greatly enjoyed by the majority of people. Familiarization is an essential part of the process. Having a bad experience early on can put people off video for good. Conversely, if the initial session is enjoyable, they will be motivated to carry on.

How the project begins consequently has a significant bearing on its success. The aim is to put the group at ease as soon as possible. The following practical steps help to ensure that this process goes smoothly.

### *Set up activities that involve everyone in front of the camera together*

Familiarization is assisted when the first few exercises involve the whole group appearing on video together (Figure 3.1). This results in everyone seeing themselves played back on screen at the same time. It does not prevent embarrassment, but at least participants undergo the ordeal together. In fact, going through the process as a group generates a sense of shared experience and solidarity, and any uncomfortable feelings soon subside.

### *Be specific about what participants say and do in front of the camera*

Once the camera is switched on, and the equipment is recording, it is much harder to think of something to say. Even quite outgoing and articulate people can dry up. For this reason give participants something simple and precise to say

49

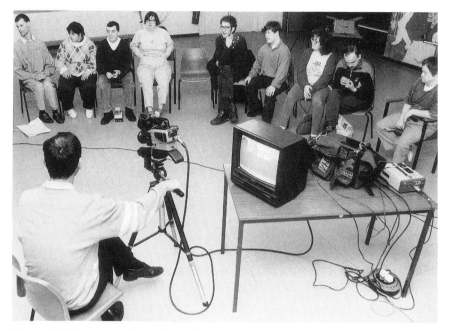

*Figure 3.1* Group introducing themselves to camera

and do on camera, particularly at the beginning. Also help them to prepare before recording starts, and prompt them if they get stuck.

## Use a hand-mike

A hand-mike is used to record sound in all the early exercises (page 260). It provides a tangible physical link between the activity in front of the camera and that behind.

The person who holds the mike is in control. Each participant is the centre of attention for a time because everyone has a turn with it, and the entire group contributes to the recorded material.

Additionally, the mike indicates whose turn it is to speak, and focuses attention on them so that the camera operator knows who to get in shot. This discourages group members from all talking at once or interrupting, because the mike cuts out sound beyond a certain distance, so that only the person holding it can be heard properly when the tape is played back.

## *Acknowledge any embarrassment after playback*

People normally feel embarrassed when they first see themselves on video. They react in a variety of ways, sometimes quite dramatically. Many laugh uproariously; others look away, or even rush out of the room. Do not hurry this process, and allow space for any response.

After the first exercise discuss how the group felt about watching themselves by finding out who has seen themselves on tape before, and asking whether anyone felt uncomfortable. Leave plenty of time for them to acknowledge any discomfort and admit to feeling embarrassed yourself to show that this is normal. Most people are noticeably relieved to find that others are feeling the same way.

It is essential to be supportive. Many participants will dislike the way they look or sound, and be critical of their performance (often reacting more to the sound of their voice than to their image). Counter any negative comments with positive feedback to build up confidence about the way they appear.

Although the whole experience is strange, most people are, at the same time, completely fascinated by watching themselves on the monitor. After a while, video playback becomes a more ordinary event, and the associated feelings recede. The group then begin to appreciate fully the video material produced.

## TYPICAL INTRODUCTORY SESSION

This section presents a typical introductory workshop, going through a series of familiarization games in the order that they are generally used. It illustrates practically how the early work develops and outlines why the games are of value.

### Preparation

To run this initial session you need to know how to do the following with the equipment (see Chapter 9).

## *Basics*

- How to wire up the equipment for use on mains power.
- How to use the video equipment safely.
- How to white balance.

## Using the camera

- How to pan and tilt the camera using the tripod.
- How to focus the camera.
- How to use the zoom lever to adjust the shot size.
- How to frame long-shots, mid-shots and close-ups.

## Using the recorder

- How to prepare to record.
- How to start and stop recording.
- How to play back recorded tape.
- How to allow for recording time lag.
- How to set up the equipment in record mode at the right place on the tape.
- How to record one shot after another.
- How to record black on tape.

## Sound

- How to use a hand-mike.
- How to use the headphones to monitor sound.
- How to set sound levels.

Before the first session starts, the equipment and room are set up as standard (page 42). Remember to perform a test recording to make sure everything is working (page 253), and white balance the camera (page 245). Then set up the equipment in record mode ready for the first exercise (page 252).

Video is used from the very beginning of the workshop. The more time spent procrastinating, the greater the apprehension participants feel about the equipment, and the longer it takes to generate a relaxed atmosphere. All the introductions can take place through video games, so there is no need for much preamble. When the group arrives, welcome them and get them seated in the chairs. Then ask who wants to use the camera first, and start the first exercise.

## NAME GAME

Procedure

The first person, seated at one end of the row of chairs, holds the hand-mike. The camera operator lines up a mid-shot of this person. The tripod is kept loose so that the camera can move freely.

Recording starts. The first person says their name and something about themselves, e.g. 'I'm Sue and I'm wearing jeans.' The mike is passed to the next person in the row, and the camera follows. They then say their name, and something about themselves, as well as restating what the first person said, e.g. 'I'm Vikram and I like chocolate, and this is Sue and she's wearing jeans.' This process continues along the row. Everyone in turn introduces themselves, and repeats all that has been said before them.

After the last person has spoken, the camera is switched off. The camera operator rewinds the tape (Figure 3.2), and the group watches the recording.

*Average time – 10 minutes*

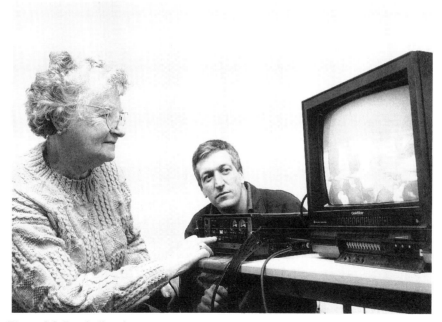

*Figure 3.2* Rewinding the tape

## Value

- *Specific task*   Participants are given something easy to say the first time on camera. The memory element further distracts them from the camera's presence.
- *Self-expression*   Group members say something introductory about themselves.
- *Appearing on video*   Everyone but the camera operator performs in front of the camera, and watches themselves played back on the monitor.
- *Group development*   The participants learn each other's names and something about one another. Going through the recording experience together develops group trust.
- *Equipment operation*   One person learns how to use the camera, and everyone else practises with the hand-mike.

## Workers' hints

The activity leader explains the game and how to use the hand-mike, whilst the technical worker introduces the camera to the camera operator. Help the camera operator set up a mid-shot (page 264), ensure that they keep the tripod loose, and help them pan along the line to cover each person speaking (page 246).

The activity leader takes part in the game. If participants are unsure about what to say, make suggestions, and if they get stuck, prompt them. The memory element of the game should not become competitive. If anyone forgets what was said, encourage the others to help them remember.

The technical worker joins in the game at the end of the row. If the camera operator is not ready to be left, the activity leader takes over the technical support role when the technical worker sits down.

Ensure that everyone learns the camera operator's name as they are the only person not to have appeared in front of the camera.

Remember to discuss how people felt about seeing themselves, especially if it is their first time on video.

After discussion, turn the monitor round, and the sound down. Reset the equipment in record mode, get someone new on the camera, and go straight on with the second game.

The name game started the process of self-expression. The next step is for the participants to find out more about each other.

Formulating questions is an essential communication skill, yet it is something that a lot of people find difficult. Those from institutionalized settings in particular are often not used to asking questions, and lack the skills required to do so.

Questioning is a very important part of video work. In a sense, every time a video programme is made it asks and answers a question. Learning how to question is fundamental to the participatory approach, and is consequently introduced early on in the familiarization process.

The following game stimulates interaction by introducing the group to the practice of forming and asking a question.

## QUESTIONS IN A ROW

### Procedure

While the camera operator learns how to use the camera, and lines up the shot, all the other participants prepare a question to ask.

The camera starts recording. Beginning at one end of the row, each person in turn uses the hand-mike to ask their question to, and receive a reply from, the person next to them. Then they hand the mike on. At the end of the row recording stops.

The exercise is rewound and played back.

*Average time – 10 minutes*

### Value

- *Communication*    Participants ask and answer questions, and get to know a bit more about each other.
- *Appearing on video*    Group members are given a specific task to perform on video together.
- *Confidence and self-worth*    Self-assurance grows through the recording and playback process, and being asked about yourself is valuing in itself.
- *Equipment use*    A new person learns how to use the camera whilst everyone else practises with the hand-mike.

### Workers' hints

Get the camera operator to set up the camera so that two people fit in the shot, starting with the first two in the row (Figure 3.3). When the camera pans along the line, the interviewer with the mike and the person answering the question should be in the picture at the same time.

Show those in front of the camera how to point the hand-mike back and forth to pick up sound between two people (page 260).

The extent to which the workers intervene to help the participants formulate

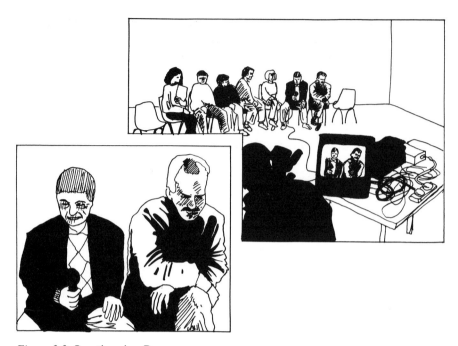

*Figure 3.3* Questions in a Row

questions depends on the individuals in the group. Give them space to try, but if they are stuck, support them.

Some people get quite confused about planning a question and then waiting until the game starts to ask it. If this is the case, just explain the game procedure, start the game, and, if necessary, help individuals think of questions in turn during recording.

The first time this game is played participants often repeat the question that they were asked, and so the same question is asked in turn down the line. Do not worry. Next time the group will have more idea what is expected, and as the project develops their questioning skills will improve.

The technical worker sits down near the end of the row to give the last participant someone to question. The activity leader can take over with the camera operator.

After playback ask the group if they found asking questions difficult, and if appropriate discuss the importance of planning. Remember that this is the first time that the camera operator from the name game has seen themselves on video.

So far in the session participants have spoken in front of the camera and have found out something about one another. They have seen themselves on tape and had some experience with the equipment. The next game encourages greater self-expression and group interaction, and develops team work.

Two additional video production roles are introduced at this stage: sound recordist and floor manager (Figure 3.4).

The sound recordist monitors the sound on the headphones (page 249). It is their responsibility to ensure that the people on camera can be heard loudly and clearly enough. The headphones focus the sound operator on the sound being recorded. Listening to them completely absorbs their attention initially, as it markedly changes their perception of the environmental sound.

At this stage sound levels can be set automatically. With some equipment it is possible to set sound levels manually (page 249). Later on in the project the sound recordists can set the levels themselves. (If the group members are particularly quick they can take on this job straight away.)

The floor manager co-ordinates the action so that everybody knows when recording has started. First they check that the camera operator, sound recordist and performers are ready to begin. Next they count three–two–one, and the camera operator starts recording. Leaving a few seconds to allow for recording time lag (page 254), they then cue the action.

Getting the group used to this simple convention from the beginning helps

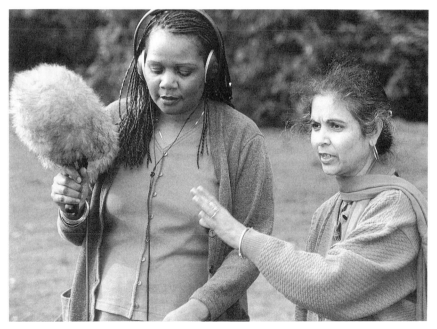

*Figure 3.4* Sound recordist and floor manager

enormously. A consistent procedure enables the group to co-ordinate their work even in the most chaotic situations.

## CHAT SHOW

### Procedure

Divide the participants into smaller groups. Three people is an ideal size. Each group picks a topic and plans two or three questions to ask. One person can be the chat show host and ask all the questions, or each person in the group can put one of the questions to the others.

Each chat show is recorded one after the other. The first group to perform decides where to sit, while another group acting as technical crew sets up the equipment: operating the camera, monitoring sound and counting in. The remaining participants play the audience.

The first chat show is recorded. Then each group swaps round, and the process is repeated. Swapping continues until each group has performed and operated the equipment.

The tape is rewound, and the chat shows are watched one after the other (Figure 3.5).

*Average time – 30–40 minutes*

### Value

- *Group development*  Up until now all interaction has been facilitated by the workshop leaders. This exercise provides the opportunity for participants to work on their own in smaller groups.
- *Communication*  Participants are stimulated to share experiences and discuss ideas within the smaller group because the topics chosen are based on their interests.
- *Individual expression*  The preceding exercises are quite structured. This task allows participants to express themselves with greater freedom.
- *Planning*  Group members prepare before recording.
- *Interviewing*  Participants develop their questioning skills and practise interviewing.
- *Production skills*  More of the group members use the camera, and sound recording and floor-managing roles are introduced.
- *Co-operation*  Team work develops as the participants work together as a technical crew, and plan and perform the chat show.

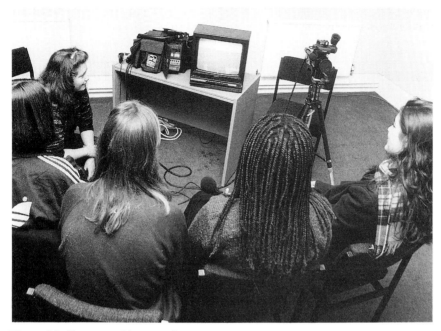

*Figure 3.5* Group watching exercise

## Workers' hints

Group members get to know each other a little more during this exercise. A relaxed mood should be encouraged. Check with each smaller group that they understand what they have to do, and then leave the room, or go out of earshot, to avoid appearing to be eavesdropping. This also demonstrates your confidence in their ability to devise something on their own.

After a while check on each group's progress and offer help with topics and question planning if required. Encourage everyone to contribute. Some groups find planning much easier than others. In some cases it may be necessary for a worker to stay with each group, facilitate the process, and take part alongside them in the chat show.

Be flexible about preparation time, but do not let it take too long. At this stage it is more important for participants to learn by going through the planning and recording process than to prepare a perfect set of questions. Five to ten minutes is usually sufficient.

Restricting each group to two or three questions helps to prevent the chat show from becoming over-long. Even so, interaction can still expand during recording. Intervene if a group goes on for a very long time, but remember that part of the purpose of this game is to get the novelty of performing on camera out of the group's system. Participants may sing, shout, dance or let off steam in other ways. If you are too rigid at this point, they may never settle down to more structured work.

One worker works with the camera operator, whilst the other organizes the sound recordist, the floor manager, the seating and the audience. Get the audience to react or clap to create a bit of atmosphere.

Encourage the performers to think about where they are going to sit. For continuity reasons, suggest that each group performs in a different place. It looks a bit odd if they pop up in the same chairs (see next game).

Remember to set up the equipment in record mode at the beginning of the exercise. If it seems appropriate, get the floor manager to do this.

If the equipment is left in record mode too long (two to five minutes, depending on equipment), it will step down (page 253). If you do not notice that record mode has disengaged, nothing will be recorded when the camera is switched on. At this early stage keep an eye on the equipment yourself. Later in the project the sound recordist can confirm that recording has started by checking that the tape is going round in the recorder. If planning is taking some time, use the standby mode to lock the equipment in record mode at the right place on the tape (page 255).

To make the recording look neater, record five seconds of black before and after each chat show (page 255).

After playback it may be appropriate to give some additional information about getting the best results from the hand-mike. Interrupt during the exercise only if there is no sound at all being recorded, not just to improve sound quality. This is only an exercise after all, and participants need a little experience going through the recording process before they are ready to consider technical improvements.

If someone asks why they cannot be heard, it is appropriate to tell them, but do not pick out someone who has used the mike badly as an example (page 231). Instead, indicate what has been done well to illustrate the point.

The Disappearing Game ends the typical introductory session. It involves using the video equipment to make people appear and disappear on tape. This effect is used on television; finding out how it is created adds to the game's appeal.

If there are six participants in the group, one will have used the camera during the Name Game, one during Questions in a Row; and if there are three smaller groups, three during the Chat Show. The last person uses the camera during this game. If there are seven in the group, swap the camera operator half way through, to make sure everyone gets a turn. If there are more people you may have to play Questions in a Row twice, or add an additional game.

## DISAPPEARING GAME

### Procedure

The camera operator sets up a wide shot showing the rest of the group sitting on chairs in a line. The tripod is then tightened so that the camera cannot be moved during recording.

The floor manager instructs everyone to keep still, and counts in. The camera is switched on, three to four seconds are recorded, and then it is switched off again.

One person leaves the scene. Everyone else stays in the same position. The floor manager co-ordinates the action, and another short shot is recorded. This process continues, one person leaving the shot each time. The empty chairs are recorded, and then everyone comes back one by one.

Rewind and playback to see participants disappear and appear (Figure 3.6).

*Average time – 20 minutes*

### Value

- *Fun*   This game often causes great hilarity, and creates a definite sense of group achievement.
- *Motivation and co-operation*   The importance of the floor manager becomes obvious. Participants can easily move when they should be still if they do not pay attention. Once the group has watched the effect, they often want to repeat the game to improve the result. Used in a chaotic setting this can instil some order, motivating participants to work as a team to co-ordinate the action.
- *Setting up shots*   Previously the camera was switched on at the start of an exercise and off at the end. This game introduces the process of deciding on a shot, setting it up, and then recording it (page 253).
- *Putting shots together*   The group record one shot after another on the tape to make a complete sequence (page 254).
- *Sense of time*   The final sequence is quite short, yet it took a while to record. This illustrates how long video takes to produce.
- *Equipment usage*   The remaining participants use the camera.

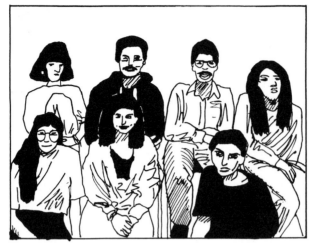

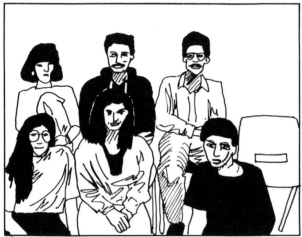

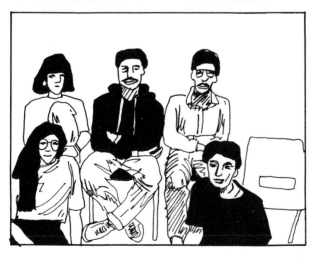

*Figure 3.6* Consecutive shots in the Disappearing Game

## Workers' hints

The best way of explaining this game is to do it. Do not get drawn into long and confusing explanations about what will happen. Just tell the group that they are going to use the equipment to make people appear and disappear, and be quite directive to ensure success.

Remember to put the equipment in record mode before the start of the exercise, and record five seconds of black at the start and end of the exercise.

If the room is small, the camera frame may not be able to accommodate the whole group sitting in a row, even when the camera is zoomed right out. If so, half the participants can stand behind the chairs, or sit on the floor at the front.

It is important that there is absolutely no camera movement at the cut between one shot and the next. Any slight shake alerts the watcher to the cut, and reduces the game's effectiveness. Ensure that the camera operator stands well back from the camera, once they have set up the shot and tightened the tripod, so that their body movements are not picked up, and get them to switch on and off carefully so that they do not jar the camera.

The effect is most striking if everyone in the picture keeps still during recording. The floor manager must co-ordinate the action so that everyone knows when the equipment is switched on. It is effective if participants maintain the same position between one shot and the next, so that only the person who leaves the shot changes. The first time the game is played this is difficult, because participants have not yet seen the effect and do not understand why they need to stay still. If the game is repeated, they will improve.

The floor manager makes sure that everyone is ready and then counts the camera in. Next they silently time the shot, and finally they cue the camera operator to switch off. They must remember to allow for recording time lag (page 254). For example, if the required shot length is three seconds, and the recording time lag is two seconds, they count five seconds before cueing the end of recording.

Timing is crucial to the game, so one of the workers should time the shot initially. If it is appropriate for a participant to take over, stand with them to make sure that they do not rush the count.

Sound is not needed for the game, so switch the microphone off or play back the tape with the monitor turned down.

If two people need to use the camera, swap at the half-way point when only the chairs are in shot, and get them to focus and reset the shot.

The final recorded piece is quite short, and usually warrants a second viewing.

This exercise generates a high point to finish the workshop. Afterwards provide time for questions and feedback, then clarify any arrangements for next time and wind up the session. Finally, ask the group to help to pack up the equipment and carry it out. Both workers should ensure that everyone has something to do, and that packing up is not dominated by one or two people.

This combination of activities provides an ideal taster session. It includes a variety of aspects of the work. All the participants use the camera, practise with the hand-mike and appear on video. The other primary production roles are introduced, and the group development process is begun, with some basic self-expression, group interaction, interviewing and team building. And of course the group has some fun – a vital component of familiarization.

Normally this session takes one to one and a half hours. If you are familiar with the equipment and the process, and working with an energetic group, it can take as little as 45 minutes; with a group that needs a slower pace it may take two hours.

## STANDARD GAME FRAMEWORKS

In a participatory video project, particular activities are often employed several times. Although the same organizational and technical procedures are repeated, the changed content and emphasis produces a different outcome according to the group's stage of development. The games and exercises outlined in the typical introductory session embody standard procedural frameworks that are used throughout the work. The following game provides another standard game framework that can be played repeatedly during a project.

### STATEMENTS IN A ROUND

## Procedure

As with the Name Game, the camera operator lines up a mid-shot of the person sitting, holding the hand-mike, at one end of the row. The tripod is kept loose, so that the camera can be moved freely.

Recording starts. The person with the mike makes a statement on a pre-arranged topic, and hands the mike on. The camera pans to the next person, who in turn makes their statement. This continues until the end of the row. Recording stops, and the tape is played back.

*Average time – 10 minutes*

## Value

- *Everyone contributes*  This game strategy can be compared to rounds in group work, where the group sits in a circle, and each person in turn makes a statement starting in a pre-arranged way. In the same way this video game creates space for the whole group to contribute. It is used to start and end sessions, to develop new ideas and to evaluate experiences.
- *Self-expression and validation*  All group members express their feelings and concerns and order their thoughts. Each person's statement is equally valued.
- *Group development*  Group members learn to listen to and respect each other's opinions. They exchange views, share experiences and develop ideas.
- *Group solidarity*  Everyone appears in front of the camera together, so no one is put on the spot. Mutual trust and group identity is developed.
- *Record of ideas*  The tape stores each person's contribution for future reference.
- *Familiarization*  Participants use the camera, speak in front of the equipment, and see themselves on video.

## Workers' hints

While the camera is set up the activity leader helps the group to prepare. If an individual has nothing to say on a subject, they can report this to camera during recording.

Do not forget that the workers should take part and make statements as well as the participants.

The main purpose of the exercise is that everyone has an input on camera. The concern is more with individual expression, the development of ideas and group awareness than the technical standard of the end-product. The floor manager can count in from their chair, and the sound recordist can set up the sound and then sit down and join in.

The camera operator is the only person not to make a statement. Include them at the end. Either get them to speak from behind the camera during recording, or video them separately before playback.

## Game variations

All the standard game frameworks can be varied to change the emphasis. The variations below illustrate how they can be adapted and repeated to different effect through the development process.

### Name Game

- *Drop the memory element of the game*    Participants start by simply saying their name in turn. Afterwards they can repeat the exercise, each saying something about themselves. Later in the process the memory aspect can be introduced. This gradual approach is suitable for special needs groups and those with limited language skills.
- *Adapt to start subsequent sessions*    With or without the memory element, participants are instructed to say something specific about themselves in turn, such as their favourite food or their hobby. This is a good way of bringing the group together at the beginning of a workshop, as it refamiliarizes them with the video process.

### Questions in a Row

- *Adapt to use at the start of subsequent sessions*    As with the Name Game, this exercise can be employed at the beginning of the workshop to remind the group what video work involves. It puts everyone in the mood, reacclimatizing them to the video workshop environment.
- *Employ to practise question asking*    Repeating the game frequently through the project improves participants' interviewing skills. It is a quick and easy way for everyone to practise asking and answering questions, and gives the workers the chance to assess how they are developing.
- *Use to find out what everyone thinks*    Each person asks the same question to the person next to them. For instance, 'Where shall we video today?', or 'What do you like about this place?' This generates input from all the participants in a way that an open question to the group does not.
- *Use to initiate discussion on a particular subject or issue*    Everyone asks a question to the person next to them on the pre-decided theme. This enables a subject to be explored, by creating the opportunity for all the participants to contribute in turn. After each person has spoken up on a subject once they are more likely to participate in an open discussion.
- *Adapt to practise question planning*    Each member of the group thinks of

a question, possibly on a pre-decided topic, and writes it on a card. The cards are shuffled, and each person picks one to ask the person next to them.

## Chat Show

The Chat Show has a very simple basic framework that works on many levels and it can be utilized again and again in different forms. Working in small groups makes it easier for everyone to participate and express their point of view.

- *Use to find out interests or concerns*   Playing the Chat Show can explore the participants' motivations and provide ideas to work on later in the project.
- *Use to explore an issue or idea*   The Chat Show provides a relaxed way of initiating discussion on a particular subject and of encouraging the group to explore and develop their opinions.
- *Play to develop group identity and cohesion*   Smaller groups provide a more intimate environment for participants to investigate shared experiences and feelings.

## Disappearing Game

This game can be adapted in numerous ways. Below are some suggestions, but experiment and see what the group members come up with.

- *Use a prop*   A hat, book or any other prop can be worn or held, and moved from person to person, or to a new position in the room, in each shot.
- *Move the group around in the frame*   For example, the group can walk, one step each shot, across the screen, or individuals can move from one position to another.
- *Play a version of Simon Says*   In each shot everyone does the same new action. For instance, they all put their arms in the air, then all sit down, then all cover their faces, and so on.
- *Represent emotions*   In a similar way the group represents emotions. For example, everyone looks sad in the first shot, then angry in the second, then happy in the next, changing their expression in each shot.
- *Transform people*   In each shot swap one person for another.
- *Objects*   Move things round, and make them appear and disappear, instead of people.
- *Create a story line*   Make each shot follow on from the next to tell a story.

Remember the Disappearing Game is at its most effective if only one thing changes in each shot. If there are lots of alterations, the effect is diluted. Build up the changes step by step for the best results.

### Statements in a Round

There are many variations to this game. It is used at the start of a session to bring the group together, and at the end to round it off. It is a simple way to get the group to begin talking about themselves and to listen to each other. It is also used to introduce a topic and develop opinions.

- *Getting to know each other*   Each person introduces themselves to the group. They make general comments or say something on a theme, such as families, friends or holidays.
- *Personal news*   Everyone says what they have done since the last session, or the best thing that has happened during the time. If you include a round of bad news, follow it by a round of good experiences.
- *Dislikes and likes*   The group plays any of the following rounds combinations:
    'I dislike . . .', followed by 'I like . . .'
    'I object to . . .', followed by 'I'm pleased that . . .'
    'I resent . . .', followed by 'I appreciate . . .'
- *Feelings*   This version can begin with a brainstorm of different feelings, or the leader can decide on a particular feeling to explore. Rounds follow such as 'I feel embarrassed when . . .', or 'I was embarrassed when . . .'. Alternatively, a round can start, 'At the moment I feel . . .'.
- *Plans and evaluation*   Rounds can encourage everyone to contribute to planning and evaluation. For example, 'I want . . .', 'I wish . . .', 'I'm here because . . .', 'I think we should . . .'; or, 'I learned . . .', 'I discovered . . .', 'I enjoyed . . .'. If you use a negative round such as 'I didn't like . . .', follow it with a positive round to end on an optimistic note.

## EXPRESSION

The games and exercises covered so far are all concerned with developing self-expression. Expression is the second stage of the participatory video process. During this stage in the work the goal is to cultivate the participants' belief that they have something worth saying, to develop their confidence to express themselves freely, and to stimulate their creativity. They are encouraged to explore, develop and verbalize their experiences, knowledge, feelings and opinions.

Some groups are fluent and articulate right from the start, and progress quickly to the next stage in the process. Other participants may have low self-esteem, little conviction that what they have to say is of value, and no previous opportunity to develop their ability to express their thoughts. Progression is slower, but is essential to their development.

Actively listen to all that the participants say, in order to build confidence in their ideas and the way they perform. Ensure that everyone has the opportunity to speak. Asking questions will generate interest in what other people have to say. Develop support and respect within the group by encouraging members to listen to one another.

Recording participants on video provides the opportunity for reflection. Matters that arise can be discussed, or referred to later in the project. However, the most important goal during the expression phase of development is that the participants become relaxed when speaking on tape. The product on tape is not the main concern and the only audience is the group themselves.

# Initial contact checklist

*Familiarization*

- Put the group at ease by using ice-breaking games.
- Establish the ground rules carefully.
- Set up games so that everyone appears in front of the camera together.
- Give participants specific tasks to do on camera.
- Use a hand-mike.
- Allow space for reactions after playback, and leave time to discuss any embarrassment.
- Do not rush this stage in the process.

*Introductory sessions*

- Use the equipment from the very start.
- Make sure that the session is enjoyable and relaxed.
- Build confidence through progressive tasks.
- Create the opportunity for self-expression.
- Introduce questioning and use it to practise with the hand-mike.
- Develop team work, and use small groups to generate communication and interaction.
- Encourage preparation and planning.
- Include sound recording and floor managing.
- Make sure roles are rotated each exercise and that everyone uses the camera during the session.
- Leave enough time to view material and for feedback and discussion.

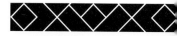

*Expression*

- **Develop participants' ability to express themselves.**
- **Get participants to practise speaking in front of the camera.**
- **Build self-esteem.**
- **Explore ideas and opinions.**
- **Discuss experiences and feelings.**
- **Concentrate on stimulating self-expression rather than on technical quality.**

Chapter 4

# Playing games

## GAMES FOR ADULTS

It is widely recognized that children use play to learn language, practise cognitive skills and rehearse social interaction as well as to re-enact and interpret difficult experiences. Adults too can benefit from the opportunity to explore their capacities in a non-threatening environment, away from daily pressures. Games are a form of structured play. Valuable learning takes place through enjoyable activity defined by a set of rules. Games can be competitive, resulting in only the most able winning at the expense of other players. They can also be co-operative, validating all participants equally, and building mutual support within the group. Group leaders use co-operative games to help participants to get to know each other, to establish rapport and to develop team spirit.

Co-operative games play an important role in the participatory video approach. Much of the project activity involves group members taking part in exercises based on simple and flexible rules. These games are valuable in participatory video projects for the reasons outlined below.

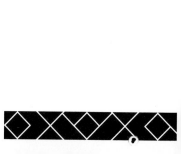

## Games are fun and help participants to relax

Video can be quite threatening if approached in a serious, critical or objectifying way. It is always strange to see and hear yourself on tape, but it can be excruciatingly embarrassing if you are being judged on your performance.

Playing games on video feels more comfortable. It creates a light-hearted and reassuring atmosphere, and can be highly entertaining. An important factor is the sense of solidarity generated by going through an unusual experience with other people. Using a games-orientated approach, participants generally find watching themselves inherently funny, and the laughter draws them closer together.

## Games stimulate participation and active involvement

Games provide the opportunity to learn through doing. Active learning is more enjoyable than lectures or demonstrations. It is also more effective because what is learnt with pleasure is less likely to be forgotten. A practical context is particularly important for acquiring the technical skills involved in video production.

## Games provide a social context in which communication and interaction can be practised in safety

Games can assist personal and social development. They are not literal, so themes and difficulties can be explored without fear of the consequences, yet the group environment generates genuine social interaction.

Games are enjoyable, but they can deal with serious matters and be revealing. A relaxed approach allows issues to be raised that may be difficult to deal with more directly. Opening up in safety creates group trust and a sense of belonging.

## Games offer flexibility to the group development process

Games can be integrated into an overall development plan, to accomplish different outcomes at different stages. The same game can be applied to break the ice, or later to achieve a particular aim. Games have an obvious use in the initial work, but they are important throughout a project. Sometimes a game is just what is needed to rekindle enthusiasm or to give insight into a new direction.

Despite their versatility, games do not provide a magic formula. All too often they are chosen to occupy a group thought incapable of more serious work, or when workers lack the skill or time to be more constructive. Games are a work tool. Each one has a range of benefits and should be played for a reason.

Clearly not all games are appropriate in all circumstances, yet be warned about generalizing about a game's suitability for a particular type of group. Fun is as good for adults as it is for young people, if not more so. Adults can need play to make connections with each other. Even if they feel initially inhibited, this soon passes, and games can also lead to important discussion. On the other hand, children, even when playing with energy and laughter, can be as incisive and serious as any adult, and often more aware.

The best games are those that fit the situation. Do not be scared about changing accepted formats if the need arises. Games are flexible, and the rules should be adapted according to the setting. In fact many of the video games in this book were developed for video from other games, to fulfil a specific function. Frequently they were devised to meet a particular need for a specific group, although all of them have been used successfully in a wide range of situations.

Game sources have been wide and diverse. Some are based on traditional children's games, some on group games in general usage, and others adapted to video from other disciplines. As they have grown over the years, they have been modified, and have evolved and matured. It is now hard to acknowledge original sources, but *Gamesters' Handbook* (Brandes and Phillips 1977) and *Video with Young People* (Dowmunt 1987) are particularly useful.

## GENERAL APPROACH

Chapter 2 covered the general participatory video approach and Chapter 3 went through a selection of video games in order to clarify the practice. The working methods outlined apply throughout the participatory video process. This means that the ground rules, and the standard working practices, both organizational and technical, apply to all the games in the book unless otherwise specified. Remember to ensure that:

- Sessions are carefully planned and structured.
- All participants have equal access to the process.
- Participants use the equipment themselves throughout.
- Roles are rotated every exercise, and all participants use the camera each session.
- Everyone present appears in front of the camera.
- One worker facilitates the technical procedure, while the other organizes the action in front of the camera.

- Games are used involving the whole group appearing on camera together at the start of each session.
- All material recorded is played back after the game.
- There is enough time for discussion.

At the start of each subsequent session the group helps to carry in the equipment and set it up, as well packing it away at the end. Participants' confidence will grow in proportion to the amount of experience they get of handling the equipment themselves. In addition, the more they are entrusted with the equipment, the more responsible they become.

Each game described follows the standard exercise procedure unless otherwise instructed. Participants' technical abilities develop through the sessions. As their skills grow, add new challenges, expect higher standards, and provide them with additional operational detail (Chapter 9). Each individual in the group will require different support, so the technical worker should respond to needs on a one-to-one basis.

At this stage it may be appropriate to get one of the group to set the equipment in record mode before each exercise (page 252) and to turn the monitor round and the sound down after playback (page 43). The sound operator can adjust sound levels manually (page 249), and the floor manager can take greater organizational responsibility as the work progresses. As many participants as feasible should be actively involved in videoing, so assign new production roles when relevant (page 139).

The games in this chapter require the same operational knowledge as Chapter 3. In addition, for particular games you need to know:

- How and when to use different microphones (pages 259–62).
- How to audio-dub (page 256).
- About lighting (pages 258–99).

After the first session the work continues to develop according to the project goals. The specific activity in each workshop depends on many factors.

Every game described is a tool to utilize during the participatory video process. Each one can generate a range of outcomes depending on the group's interests, stage of development and the subject matter. Many of them, like those already covered, provide generalized frameworks for group video work and can be used several times in the process to different effect.

Video games develop technical skills and understanding of the medium; co-operation and team work; expression, interaction and communication; the participants' ideas; and representation of their point of view on video. Social and technical skills evolve in parallel, through the process. The emphasis in a game usually depends on precisely what is needed at that moment in the project.

Nonetheless, for ease of reference, they have been categorized according to their primary purpose.

The games in this chapter are divided into those that look specifically at the nature of the medium, and those that aim predominantly for individual or group development. The average time needed to play each game is also given as a guide to aid planning.

## MEDIUM-BASED GAMES

This section covers games that investigate the nature of the video medium. They are divided into five categories: framing games, media education games, miming games, sound games and camera-effect games. They all develop technical skills, and a greater understanding of video, as well as continuing the group development process.

## Framing games

The frame is the rectangular picture area created by the camera that defines what can be seen in the shot. Framing is the process by which the camera is moved and zoomed in and out to create the frame. The subject size in the shot, in relation to the picture area, is adjusted during framing. If tightly framed, the subject fills most of the picture; if loosely framed, there is more space round the subject (page 263).

Several games consider the frame, and practise framing.

### HEADS, HANDS AND FEET

Introduces the concept of the frame experientially.

### Procedure

Initially, one of the workers operates the camera. Define a frame area by panning the camera, and zooming in or out, then tighten the tripod. Position the monitor so that the whole group can see the screen. Ask the participants to place a number of parts of the body in the frame, so that they can be seen on the monitor, e.g. 'Can I have three feet in the picture?'

Group members step forward, and move until there are three feet, and only feet, on the screen (Figure 4.1).

Each turn the camera is repositioned and the process is repeated for other requests: such as two heads, one wheelchair wheel, or twelve fingers. Every time participants must move until the screen is filled accordingly. After a few rounds one of the group uses the camera, and makes suggestions. Pointing the camera at difficult angles may mean climbing on chairs, or lying on the ground. Swapping continues until everyone has had several turns in front of the camera.

*Average time – 15 minutes*

## Value

- *Frame awareness*   The group explores the space defined by the camera in the wider environment where the game is taking place. They discover where it is in relationship to the camera, and how it changes according to distance.
- *Co-operation*   Participants work together to find the frame in the room space, and to discover how to fill it completely without blocking each other.
- *Movement*   The game involves standing up and moving around. It generates activity if the group have been still for some time.
- *Camera operation*   The camera operator considers the space needed for the parts of the body requested, and practises setting up the camera to create a suitable frame.

## Workers' hints

Clear the room and move everyone to one side, so that there is plenty of room to create an empty frame.

This game breaks convention in that one of the facilitators uses the camera initially. (Present it as the worker's turn.) This ensures that the frame is appropriate for the request. (Asking for four feet and pointing the camera at the ceiling will not work.) After a few rounds have been played, it is clear what is expected, and a group member can take over. One worker stays with them, whilst the other helps those in front to move to fill the picture.

Turn the monitor towards the action so that those in the picture can see what they are doing. (If the camera changes direction, this can mean changing the way the monitor faces each turn.) Point out what is happening on the screen to encourage participants to use it for feedback.

The frame defines a space that is three-dimensional rather than two-dimensional. This space is cone-shaped, emanating from the camera lens. The further away an object is from the camera, the more can fit into the picture (Figure 4.1). Get people to explore the effect of distance by moving closer if they need to be bigger, as well as laterally to move out of the frame edge.

Using the monitor for feedback can be surprisingly confusing. People expect it to be like a mirror. It isn't. If you move your left hand, it is on the right side as you look at the monitor. Help participants to understand which way they need to move in relation to the screen image.

Encourage the more reserved group members to take part. Ensure that everyone swaps round, making sure that the same people do not appear in every shot. Remember that the workers should also take part in front of the camera.

It is not necessary to record this exercise to get benefit from it. However, it can be turned into a version of the Disappearing Game by recording a few seconds of each frame, one shot after another. This provides additional recording practice.

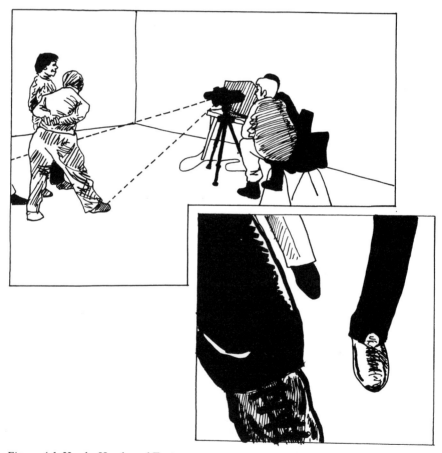

*Figure 4.1* Heads, Hands and Feet

## Variations

- *Request items from the room*  For example, two hats, one chair or three pencils.
- *Explore the edge of frame*  Ask for volunteers to hold up the roof (the top frame edge), lean on the walls (the side frame edges), or to line up items such as chairs so that they are just in the shot.
- *Develop group awareness by asking for*:
  1 Likes and dislikes. For example, all those who like chocolate, or who dislike spiders.
  2 Similarities and differences amongst group members. For example, all those with brown eyes, all those who live in a flat, or all those with a bicycle.
  3 Opinions. For example, all those who want to record a video about the locality, all those who want to do drama, or all those who think traffic should be banned from the town.

## WHO'S IN THE PICTURE?

Develops awareness of the relationship between the camera position and the shot content.

## Procedure

Turn the monitor away from the group, or cover it, so that the screen cannot be seen. The camera operator decides, without telling the group, who is to be in the shot, and frames the shot accordingly. Everyone else has to guess who is in the picture. When all group members have made a guess, the monitor is uncovered to show the shot. The camera operator then changes.

*Average time – 10 minutes*

## Value

- *Camera direction awareness*  Group members assess what is in shot by looking at where the camera is pointing.
- *Camera operation*  The camera operator practises choosing and framing a shot (Figure 4.2).
- *Involvement*  Everyone can succeed at this simple guessing game.

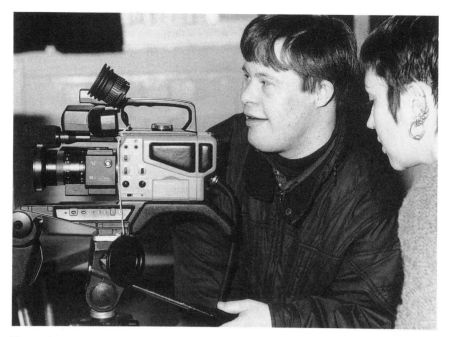

*Figure 4.2* Framing a shot

## Workers' hints

It is important that the camera operator frames the shot they choose rather than just arriving at it by accident. Get them to explain who they want in the picture, without anyone else hearing, and help them to achieve their aim.

The activity worker encourages the rest of the group to work out where the camera is pointing by looking at the lens. Stimulate guesses by asking questions, e.g. 'Where is the camera pointing? How many people are in the picture? Who's in the picture?'

## I SPY

Practises selecting potential shots, and framing in response to direction.

## Procedure

Ask who wants to be the director. The first director then chooses a shot of something in the room. They tell the group whether they want a close-up, mid-shot or long-shot, and give a clue as to the object, e.g. 'I spy with my close-up eye something blue.' The clue should be something that can be seen, such as colour, texture, size, shape or even function.

The camera operator then searches with the camera. The director tells them when they are warmer (nearer), or colder (further away). The other group members ask the director questions about the object in turn, e.g. 'Is it long? Is it used to write?' The director can answer only yes or no.

When the camera operator finds the object, they frame an appropriate-sized shot. The director ends the game when they are satisfied, and everyone swaps round.

*Average time – 20 minutes*

## Value

- *Camera control*   The camera operator frames the shot according to the director's specification, developing greater control of the camera.
- *Close observation*   The participants look at the environment carefully, seeing details that they would normally miss.
- *Decision making*   There may be hundreds of different shots in a room. Participants consider potential shots, and decide on one.
- *Being in control*   Each director controls the action for their shot.
- *Questions*   Group members practise formulating questions.

## Workers' hints

One worker takes the director aside. Ensure that they are specific about the shot, and that their clue relates to the object chosen.

Make sure that the questions are asked one at a time, and get the camera operator to stop moving and consider the answer before searching again.

When searching, ensure that the camera is not zoomed right in, as this makes it impossible to make out what is in the picture.

It is not necessary to record this exercise. However, a few seconds of each completed frame can be recorded shot by shot to provide additional recording practice.

## Media education games

Every process of relaying a message through a medium has an effect on the original message. These games encourage participants to explore the subjectivity of the process through experience.

### GRANDPARENT'S FOOTSTEPS

A video version of Grandmother's Footsteps. Generates discussion on the relationship between a recorded image and reality.

### Procedure

Set up the equipment at one end of the room. One person operates the camera and another watches the monitor. Position the monitor so that the watcher has their back to the action. Everyone else stands at the other end of room.

Recording starts and players try to creep up and touch the tripod. The camera operator attempts to catch them moving on camera. The monitor watcher sends anyone they see moving on the screen back to the beginning. The game finishes when the first person reaches the tripod, and recording ends.

Everyone swaps round, and the game is played three or four times. Then it is watched with the sound turned down.

*Average time – 20 minutes*

### Value

- *Co-operation*   If the players spread out and work together, the camera operator cannot cover everyone. The camera operator and watcher must also co-operate because, if the camera pans frantically from side to side, the watcher sees only a blur on the screen.
- *Frame-edge awareness*   Group members look at the camera direction to assess whether they are in shot.
- *Understanding the medium*   Participants move a lot in the game, and remember this experience, yet the recorded material shows predominantly motionless people because most of the action takes place off-camera. This can stimulate discussion about video as an impartial observer of reality.
- *Movement*   If the group members have been sitting around, or engaged in serious discussion for a while, the game can generate movement.
- *Numbers*   This game also works with a larger group.

## Workers' hints

Agree on a signal between the watcher and the participants so that they know if they are spotted moving.

One worker should stay with the monitor to assist the watcher and ensure fair play.

A long-shot shows all participants on the monitor all the time, and the game will not work. Make sure the camera is set up for a mid-shot or close-up (page 264), and ban the use of the zoom.

This game needs a reasonable amount of space to work. In a smaller room, restrict the size of the shot to a close-up, or reduce the size of step that players can take.

Play back enough of the game to initiate a discussion, but it may not be necessary to watch everything recorded in this case.

## VIDEO WHISPERS

Looks at the way that any transmission medium changes a message.

### Procedure

A camera operator and sound recordist set up a mid-shot of one of the workers sitting on a chair. Everyone else goes out of the room so that they cannot hear. The camera starts, and the worker tells a short story to camera, with plenty of description, and a detailed plot.

Recording stops, and roles are swapped round. The sound recordist now sits in the chair, the camera operator becomes sound recordist, and a new camera operator is called in. The group member in front of the camera then relates the story to the camera, repeating as much detail as possible. Role swapping continues until everyone has told the story.

Watch the tape to see how the story changes between the first and last version.

*Average time – 25 minutes*

### Value

• *Nature of mediated messages*  The story changes in detail through the process. The group discusses how a medium can alter a message.

83

- *Confidence in public speaking*    Each group member practises speaking alone in front of camera.
- *Listening and relating*    Participants concentrate on actively listening to the story details, memorizing them, and repeating the tale from memory.
- *Production*    As technical roles are swapped each time the story is related, everyone practises each production role.

## Workers' hints

Participants who have not told the story must remain out of earshot, otherwise someone with a good memory might go last yet remember details from the first telling.

It is hard for participants to concentrate on listening when they are operating the camera, so everyone hears the story twice, once as camera operator and once as sound recordist, before they repeat it.

Comparison between the first and the last version is most revealing. After playing back the whole exercise, watch these versions again one after the other. The story detail usually disappears, and the storyline can change completely. Discuss how any medium can corrupt a message.

A lapel mike can be introduced during this exercise (page 262). Get the sound recordist to plug it in and set it up.

## DOPPELGANGER

Explores camera angles and shot sizes.

## Procedure

The group divides into pairs. Each pair thinks of two opposite characteristics to represent, for example: important and unimportant; serious and comical; or confident and shy. Each pair decides on the camera angle, shot size, background, positioning, gestures and expressions to use to represent the two characteristics.

One member of the pair operates the camera and the other performs both characteristics. Other participants set sound levels, floor manage, and arrange the furniture and backdrop. The camera starts, and the performer expresses their first characteristic. For instance, 'I am important.' Then they set up and record the second characteristic. Swap round, and repeat for all the pairs.

*Average time – 30 minutes*

- *Understanding video* Participants explore how camera angles and shot sizes express meaning, and reflect on the way in which presentation affects representation.
- *Expression* The group experiment with body language and voice to represent qualities.
- *Group development* Working in pairs develops relationships.
- *Production skills* Everyone swaps roles repeatedly, generating lots of equipment practice.

## Workers' hints

The same member of each pair represents both of the opposite characteristics, to make the contrast between them stronger. This also means that one person does not represent the more negatively valued quality only. If there is time, get both of the pair to perform.

The game takes some time, but it teaches the group a lot about how video represents subtle meaning. Discuss how both factual and fictional programmes use camera angles.

Record five seconds of black between each shot to make the recording tidier.

## Miming games

Miming games explore how actions, gestures and facial expressions convey meaning.

## MIMED INTRODUCTIONS

A silent alternative to the Name Game.

## Procedure

Using the Name Game framework, the camera operator starts the camera. Each person in turn mimes an action, facial expression or gesture to introduce themselves. The mime can represent their personality, the way they are feeling or what they do. The camera is set up for a mid-shot, and pans along the line to cover each mime, stopping after the last person. Play back the recording.

*Average time – 15 minutes*

## OBJECT MIME

Develops non-verbal self-expression.

## Procedure

Prepare a variety of unusual objects. Set up as for the previous exercise, with the first person holding one of the objects.

The camera starts. The person mimes a use for the object, and then hands it on. The next person mimes a second use, and so on until the end of the line when the camera is switched off. Roles are swapped, and the game is repeated with the second object. After a few rounds, play back the recording.

*Average time – 15 minutes*

## Value

- *Warm-up*   These two games provide alternative ice-breakers. Participants are given something specific to do on camera, and everyone appears together.
- *Self-expression*   Group members express themselves non-verbally.
- *Trust and confidence*   Through trying something new, participants gain confidence and develop trust in one another.

## Workers' hints

Remember to leave time to acknowledge any embarrassment, particularly if these games are used early on, or if the participants are new to drama.

If necessary, help participants to prepare before recording starts. Prompt them by asking how they are feeling, or what they like doing, and get them to make suggestions to each other. The purpose is to build confidence and develop group support, not to put anyone on the spot.

Make sure that the camera operator keeps the tripod loose so that they are ready to follow any mime action.

## PASS THE COIN

Develops imagination and co-operation.

### Procedure

Everyone sits in a row apart from the camera operator and a monitor watcher. The monitor is positioned so that the watcher has their back to the group. Recording starts and a coin is passed back and forth between participants, whilst concealing its location from the camera. Participants without the coin also mime passing back and forth to confuse the watcher.

The camera operator tries to reveal the coin's position. The monitor watcher guesses where it is. When the guess is correct, recording stops, and everyone swaps round. The game is played several times. Watch the tape to see if participants can locate the coin on playback.

*Average time – 15 minutes*

### Value

- *Involvement*   Everyone is actively engaged together in a group endeavour.
- *Co-operation*   Those in front of the camera work together to conceal the coin; the monitor watcher and camera operator try to find it.
- *Technical skills*   The camera operator practises moving the camera by tilting, panning and zooming.
- *Understanding video*   Playback can generate discussion about how well the camera followed what was actually happening.

### Workers' hints

Make sure that the camera operator zooms neither all the way in so that they cannot make anything out, nor right out so that everyone is in the shot.

If the group members are very good at hiding the coin, try a larger object, or increase the gap between each chair.

## IN THAT WAY

Develops communication, social interaction and non-verbal expression.

## Procedure

Two groups are formed, and each group secretly picks an adverb. One group stands in a line in front of the camera. The other group stands in a line by the equipment. The first person in the equipment line operates the camera, and the second person holds the hand-mike.

The camera starts, and the hand-mike holder asks the first person in front of the camera to do an action in the manner of the adverb they have chosen, e.g. 'Walk in that way', or 'Get dressed in that way.' If the adverb is 'angrily', the person in front of the camera must walk, or get dressed, angrily.

Those behind the camera swap roles. The camera moves to the second person, and the new mike holder makes a second request to the second person in front of the camera. This continues until the end of the line. The camera is stopped, and the two groups swap round and repeat.

Play back and each group tries to guess the other's adverb.

*Average time – 20 minutes*

## Value

- *Creative self-expression* Those miming react spontaneously to the requests, imaginatively improvising a response.
- *Communication* Participants practise using the mike to make requests, as well as communicating non-verbally.
- *Social development* The game involves considerable interaction and co-operation between the team members.
- *Technical skills* The camera operator practises following action. Everyone co-ordinates technical role swapping.

## Workers' hints

Ensure that the camera operator does not zoom in too far; if the mime is expansive they may miss the action.

## Sound games

These games explore the relationship of sound to pictures.

### EMOTIONS

Explores how meaning can be expressed through simple facial expressions, and practises interpreting and commentating.

#### Procedure

Each person thinks of a facial expression to represent a chosen emotion, such as joy or astonishment. A commentator, using the hand-mike, watches the monitor with their back to the action. A first performer stands alone in front of the camera, if possible positioned so that they cannot hear the commentary. The camera sets up for a close-up of the performer's face.

Recording starts, the performer makes their expression, and the commentator explains what the person is feeling. Recording stops, everyone swaps round, and the next performer is recorded. Each emotion is recorded shot by shot (page 254). At the end the tape is played back, and the match between the commentary and the intended emotion is discussed.

*Average time – 15 minutes*

### COMMENTARY GAME

Practises interpreting and commentating.

#### Procedure

The set-up and procedure are the same as for the previous exercise, but this time each group member secretly decides on an activity to mime.

The camera operator starts recording. The performer mimes and the commentary begins. At the end the camera stops and everyone swaps round.

The game continues until everyone has mimed, operated the camera and spoken. The recording is then played back and the commentary compared with the mimer's chosen activity.

*Average time – 30 minutes*

## GROUP MIME

### Procedure

Two groups are formed. Each group thinks of a short story to mime. The first group mimes, while the other group operates the camera, sets the sound levels, floor manages and commentates. After recording the groups swap round and repeat. During playback the commentary is compared to the mimers' story.

The game can be developed further by audio-dubbing new commentaries on the mimes. This can improve the piece by matching the story better or dramatizing the atmosphere; or make it funnier by deliberately mismatching the commentary.

*Average time – 30 minutes*

## NEW SOUND-TRACK

Explores how sound affects the way images are read.

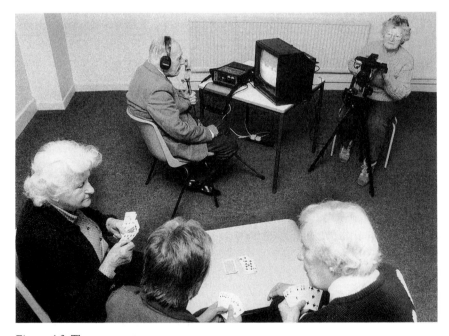

*Figure 4.3* The commentary game

## Procedure

Before the session, copy the same section of a programme onto two video tapes.

The group sets up the equipment to audio-dub a new sound-track onto one of the copies (page 256). One person sets up the recorder, another the sound levels, and a third is the floor manager.

The audio-dub can be improvised spontaneously. The recorder starts, and the mike is passed along each time a different character speaks. Alternatively, the group can prepare by watching the tape first (preferably without sound) to assign characters. Play back the original version with sound, followed by the copy with the new sound-track, and compare.

The same exercise can done with music. In this case three copies of the original piece are made. Two contrasting pieces of music are picked, and the group over-dubs them onto two of the taped copies. They are then played back to compare the effect of the music in each case.

*Average time – 30 minutes*

## Value

- *Effect of sound*   All these games investigate how sound affects meaning on video.
- *Creative expression*   The group is involved in dramatic improvisation, either spoken or non-verbal.
- *Team-work*   Each game requires that technical roles are co-ordinated and performers co-operate.
- *Sound*   Participants gain experience of setting sound levels, using micro-phones and audio-dubbing.
- *Social development*   Group members interact, represent and interpret, and develop awareness of others.

## Workers' hints

Not all video equipment can audio-dub. Check your equipment and make sure you know the procedure (page 256).

When audio-dubbing, remember to turn the monitor sound down or it will produce feedback in the way that it does when sound and pictures are recorded together (page 43).

The activity leader makes sure that everyone has a mime prepared, and helps them to think of something simple if they are stuck. Be supportive, and do not put anyone on the spot.

One of the workers stands by the commentator to prompt them, by asking questions, if they dry up.

Remember most recorded music, television programmes and pre-recorded videos are covered by copyright (page 125). You need permission to copy any material. Use original or copyright-free music and video.

## Camera-effect games

All the following games use the camera to create a special visual effect. Although the activities are slightly bizarre and the effects seem tacky, they are commonly used on television and are fun to try out.

### MOUNTAIN CLIMBING

### Procedure

The camera is turned through approximately 90 degrees on the tripod base and then resecured. It is then tipped onto its side, and pointed at the floor, so that the floor appears to be vertical on the monitor (Figure 4.4).

The camera operator starts the camera running. Participants crawl along the ground in an upwards direction on the monitor (determined, if necessary, by one worker demonstrating) and appear on screen to be climbing a vertical slope.

After watching the playback the game can be repeated with further dramatization, such as: extra effort, ropes for safety, and falls down the mountain (rolling).

### EARTHQUAKE

### Procedure

After making sure that the camera is securely attached to the tripod plate, the tripod is loosened so that it can move freely in all directions. The tripod arm is shaken up and down and from side to side. Everyone in front of the camera acts as if the floor is shaking, and jumps around, as if being thrown about. This creates an earthquake effect (Figure 4.5).

After demonstration, a scene can be dramatized. The camera starts, and everyone walks around acting normally. On a pre-arranged signal, the camera is

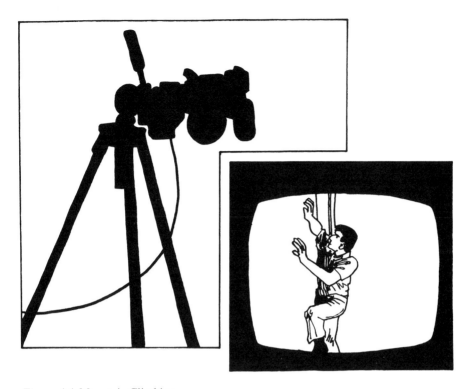

*Figure 4.4* Mountain Climbing

shaken, and everyone in shot jumps around. On another signal, the quake stops, and everyone recovers.

## STORM AT SEA

### Procedure

The camera is turned through 90 degrees on the tripod base and resecured. If the camera is tipped from side to side, it looks as if the floor is slopping one way and then the other, as if on a boat in a rough sea (Figure 4.6). Those in front of the camera move from side to side as if they were being tipped across the deck one way and the other.

After establishing which way to move, recording starts. Everything starts calm then, on a pre-arranged signal, the camera starts tipping, and people start moving. The storm builds up to a crescendo by increasing the movement, and then calms down again.

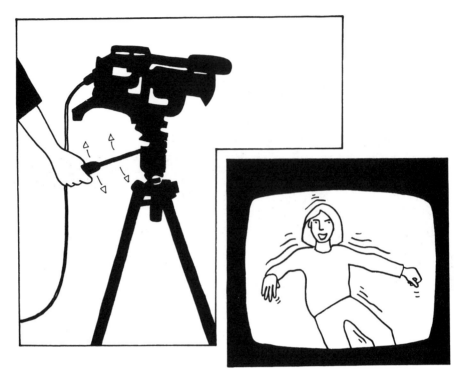

*Figure 4.5* Earthquake

## LOST IN SPACE

### Procedure

The camera is taken off the tripod. It is then moved slowly from side to side and upside down. Those in front of the camera act as if they were floating in space. After demonstration the effect can be dramatized, and recorded.

*Average time – 20 minutes*

### Value

- *Motivation*  These games involve lots of movement and are good warm-up exercises. Participants take part in an amusing activity that can also be an outlet for any excess energy.
- *Expression*  Group members are involved in imaginative dramatic inter-pretation.

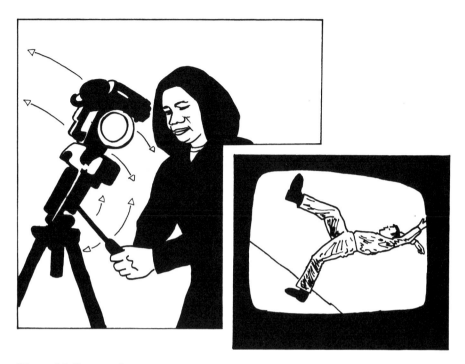

*Figure 4.6* Storm at Sea

- *Understanding television* Groups gain a better understanding of how effects are produced.
- *Group size* These games can work with large groups.

## Workers' hints

Practise all the effects before you use them with a group, to make sure the technical set-up is clear.

One worker can demonstrate the effect so that the participants understand what is expected.

Clear the area before the game. Stationary chairs on the side of the mountain, or unaffected by the earthquake, spoil the illusion.

Use lighting and props to make the background look more realistic.

Initially, play back with the monitor sound turned down.

### Development

All these camera effects can be used as the basis of the following exercise, which progressively builds up a news programme.

## ATMOSPHERE

The original recording may well have an incongruous sound-track, consisting mainly of laughter. A more appropriate sound-track can be recorded to replace the original using the audio-dub function (page 256).

## Procedure

One member of the group sets up the video recorder, one positions the mike and sets the sound levels, and one is the floor manager. Everyone else finds an object to produce a suitable sound effect. These can be instruments or objects supplied for the game, or objects found around the room. Feet can be stamped, spoons rattled in coffee cups, hands clapped, paper crackled, curtains shaken, and voices used to shout or create other vocal effects. This imitates a Foley studio where feature film sound-tracks are created.

The floor manager counts in, and the audio-dub starts. Mountain climbing can include sounds of the climbers talking, and the wind and the rain. The earthquake game could start with chatting, and turn to shouting and screaming when the quake begins.

At the end play back to see the difference the new sound-track makes to the recording.

*Average time – 20 minutes*

## Value

- *Effect of sound*   The new sound-track really alters the recording, even when the sound effects are crude and fun to produce. What was an entertaining effect becomes much more realistic, despite the backdrop. This strongly illustrates the importance of sound in creating atmosphere.
- *Audio-dub*   The group members learn how to dub a new sound-track on to pre-recorded pictures.

## Workers' hints

This exercise can be produced only on equipment that has an audio-dub facility. Make sure you understand how to use the function before trying it in a workshop (page 256). If it goes wrong the first time, simply repeat the operation, correcting any mistakes.

Alternatively, if your equipment cannot audio-dub, repeat the game with half the group creating a live sound-track, whilst the other half re-enact the scene.

## NEWS REPORT

The exercise can then be developed still further to produce an imaginary news report.

## Procedure

The original recording becomes live footage received by a news studio. The camera operator sets up a shot of a newscaster behind a desk. An introduction is recorded after the effect on the tape, e.g. 'The programme has just been interrupted by live footage being transmitted directly to the studio of a boat in trouble off the coast.' Everyone swaps roles, and interviews with those at the scene can then be recorded.

*Average time – 25 minutes*

## Value

- *Active engagement*    Although many of the camera-effect games are based on disasters, these can bring up important issues. On one occasion the earthquake was played at a youth club with 11–14 year olds. Jumping around during the quake generated lots of laughter, and everyone got carried away with tomato ketchup and toilet-paper bandages when recreating the aftermath. Then some of the survivors at the scene refused to be interviewed, confronting the crew about their right to be there. This generated important discussion about the ethics of recording people in trauma. The discussion emerged from the group's total involvement in the activity. With this approach they were led into more serious and structured work through active engagement in a light-hearted game.

  This development process is an example of how programme making can be introduced through simple stages, starting with a relatively unstructured, enjoyable game, and resulting in more organized activity addressing serious topics.

## Workers' hints

Unless the equipment you are using has a picture insert facility, it is impossible to record the news desk presentation before the live footage without erasing some of the following recording, and creating several seconds of blank tape (pages 255–6). As suggested, record the news desk, and interview shot by shot after the live footage.

## INDIVIDUAL AND SOCIAL DEVELOPMENT

The last chapter covered games to use in the initial stages of participatory video work. It concentrated on basic familiarization games and those that develop self-expression. All participatory video games are used as tools for individual and group development, but this is the primary purpose in the following games.

## Self-expression

There are many ways to stimulate the group members to talk about themselves, and express what they think, in addition to the games already described.

## OBJECTS

Uses objects to prompt expression.

## Procedure

Each person finds an object, either by searching round the room, or looking through their possessions, and then spends a few minutes examining it in close detail.

The game format is the same as for Statements in a Round. The camera starts, and each person in turn describes their object in detail. They include everything they can see about it, what it is used for, and whether its name fits its function.

Recording is stopped, and the tape watched.

*Average time – 20 minutes*

### Value

- *Expression*   People frequently find it hard to think of what to say when they are in front of the camera. The objects provide a stimulus. The game variations promote observation, improvisation, and communication of past experiences.

### Variations

- *Personal Objects*   Get each participant to bring in an object from home, and describe what it means to them, or relate a connected event in their life. This introduces oral history work.
- *Object Functions*   Collect a variety of unusual objects. The camera operator focuses on one of them. Each person in turn describes a possible use for the object, the more imaginatively the better. Swap round and repeat for the other objects.

## OPINIONS

Develops the expression of opinions.

### Procedure

Using the same game framework as Statements in a Round, each person speaks in turn about a topic they feel strongly about. The camera is switched on. Each person makes their comment, and passes the mike to the next person. Group members either talk spontaneously, or complete a statement such as, 'I feel strongly about . . . because. . . .'

Alternatively, each statement can be recorded shot by shot (page 254).

*Average time – 20 minutes*

### Value

- *Expression*   Participants are often reluctant to express strong opinions to camera. They can lack confidence in their beliefs, fearing that they are not valid, or even wrong. They may subconsciously believe that it is impolite to voice strong views. These games encourage them to verbalize their beliefs.

## Variations

- *Complaints*  First get participants to brainstorm possible grievances, such as the weather, traffic or parents. Each participant chooses a complaint from the list, or the whole group picks the same complaint.

## Community building

The following games develop interaction, mutual acceptance, trust, reflective listening and group cohesion.

## QUESTIONS IN A CIRCLE

This is a more complicated version of Questions in a Row, requiring greater co-ordination.

## Procedure

Group members sit in chairs placed in a large circle. The camera is placed in front of one of the chairs, and set up to record two people sitting in a pair of chairs at the opposite side of the circle.

The camera starts, and one of the two people asks the other a question, to which they reply. The entire group then moves round one place, resulting in a new camera operator, a new interviewer, and the person who asked the last question now replying.

The process continues until everyone has used the camera, and recording is stopped.

*Average time – 20 minutes*

## Value

- *Camera operation*  This game is excellent with larger groups, or if time is short, because it gives everyone a turn on the camera.
- *Appearing on video*  All the participants perform on camera, and watch themselves played back.
- *Communication*  Participants ask and answer questions.

## Workers' hints

As the game is quite pressurized it may not always be appropriate, especially near the start of the project, or if the group have mobility difficulties.

Hurry everyone along if the camera is kept running throughout, as described above. Alternatively, switch the camera off between questions, creating the opportunity for each camera operator to set up the shot.

## PAIRS

Cultivates group relationships.

## Procedure

Divide the group into pairs. One person in each pair spends about five minutes introducing themselves to their partner. The pair swaps round and the second person speaks. The listening partner asks questions to prompt or clarify.

The first pair sits in front of the camera. A second pair operates the camera and monitors sound. Other participants floor-manage and play the audience. Recording starts and each person introduces their partner to the group. Recording stops, the pairs swap round, and the process is repeated, continuing until each pair has performed.

*Average time – 25 minutes*

## Value

- *Group development*    Participants find out more about each other.
- *Individual development*    Through revealing and presenting themselves, self-awareness grows.
- *Active listening*    Group members concentrate on listening to each other so that they can relate what they have heard.
- *Representation*    Each person presents their partner on tape.
- *Production*    There is plenty of opportunity to practise production roles.

## Workers' hints

Encourage participants to work with someone who they do not know very well rather than sticking with a friend.

Other microphones can be introduced during the game. Try a different mike for each pair, and compare the resulting sound (pages 259–62).

## STORY CONSEQUENCES

Creates a group story.

### Procedure

Use the same game format as the Name Game. The camera starts, and the first person starts telling a story. On a pre-arranged signal (e.g. a clap), they pass the hand-mike on to the next person, who must continue the story. The story finishes at the end of the row, or the mike goes round until the story concludes. Recording stops, and the tape is played back.

*Average time – 20 minutes*

### Value

- *Creativity*   Participants improvise a storyline without pre-planning.
- *Group development*   A sense of collective achievement is generated, through group creativity.
- *Narrative*   The process of telling a story, one event after the next, is introduced.

### Workers' hints

Get each group member to add just a line or two to the story. Do not leave them talking until they flounder.

## POSITIVE FEEDBACK

Participants give and receive positive appraisal.

<h2>Procedure</h2>

Divide the participants into two groups. One group becomes the technical crew. The other group sits in front of the camera.

Recording starts and each person in turn uses the hand-mike to say something positive about all of the others in their group. The camera stops, the groups swap, and the process is repeated. The tape is then played back.

*Average time – 20 minutes*

<h2>Value</h2>

- *Group development* Through giving and receiving positive feedback, mutual support and trust is developed.
- *Self-esteem* Most people are all too able to provide negative criticism of themselves and others. Hearing constructive comments can be a strange experience, but it generates a positive self-awareness.

<h2>Workers' hints</h2>

Make sure that all the comments are positive. Encourage other members of the group to make suggestions if anyone is stuck.

## LOOKING AT OTHERS

Explores how people assess each other on first sight.

<h2>Procedure</h2>

Use the standard game set-up as for Questions in a Row. The camera operator sets up a mid-shot of the first two people in the row.

The camera starts and the first person tells the second person something that they can clearly see about them, e.g. 'It's apparent that you wear glasses.' The second person then says what they can see about the third person, and so on down the line. Recording stops, and the technical roles are swapped.

In the next round each person says something that they surmise about the person next to them, e.g. 'I imagine that you like playing sport.' This time they check out what they say by asking, 'Am I right?' Watch the tape and discuss how people are assessed on the way they appear.

*Average time – 20 minutes*

## Value

- *Awareness of assumptions*   The group members gain insight into the way they judge others on appearance.
- *Group development*   Trust and understanding is developed through communication and interaction.

## Workers' hints

In the first round participants say something that is completely obvious, such as what the person is wearing, and must not make any assumptions. During the next round participants can make guesses.

## UNDERSTANDING OTHERS

Encourages the group to explore feelings.

## Procedure

Everyone, including the workers, writes a fear on a piece of paper, e.g. 'I am afraid that if I say what I think people will think I'm stupid.' All the pieces of paper are placed in a box and shaken around. Each person then chooses one.

Using the same format as the Name Game, recording starts. Each person reads out the fear they have picked, and then expands on it to explain what the person who wrote it was feeling. Recording stops, and the tape is played back.

*Average time – 20 minutes*

## Value

- *Expression*   Participants share their feelings, and have them accepted, in relative security.
- *Awareness*   Group members develop awareness of their own and each other's feelings.

- *Group development* Through group acceptance, mutual trust and understanding is cultivated.

## Workers' hints

Make sure that the workers reveal their feelings, as well as the participants.

## Variations

- Share and acknowledge complaints, worries, wishes, or likes and dislikes.

## Communication

Many of the games in this book develop interaction amongst the participants. Using video is an effective way to stimulate communication both within the group, and between the participants and other people. As stated previously, one of the most important abilities developed through the participatory video process is that of asking questions. The following interviewing exercises all develop communication skills.

## INTRODUCING INTERVIEWS

## Procedure

The group are divided into pairs. Each pair thinks of a topic, and prepares three or four questions to ask. One partner is the interviewer, the other answers the questions.

The first two perform their interview, whilst the other participants operate the camera, set up the sound, direct, floor-manage and play the audience.

After the first interview everyone swaps round. The process is repeated until all the interviews have been recorded.

*Average time – 30 minutes*

## Value

- *Questions*  Participants practise formulating questions and interviewing.
- *Interaction*  Pairs discuss ideas, develop issues and decide how to address their topic.
- *Planning*  Everyone prepares before recording.
- *Production*  Group members swap round production roles for each interview.

## Workers' hints

Interviews are similar in format to those in the Chat Show, but always happen in pairs and are more formal. When you support the planning process, encourage participants to ask open questions (what, where, who, how, why?), rather than those that produce yes/no answers.

## IN THE HOT SEAT

## Procedure

The camera operator sets up a mid-shot of one member of the group sitting in front of the camera. Everyone else sits in a row facing them.

The camera starts. The microphone is passed along the row, and everyone asks a question to the interviewee in the hot seat. Recording stops and someone else takes a turn.

*Average time – 5 minutes to set up and 5 minutes for each person*

## Value

- *Individual development*  Participants reveal things about themselves, and self-awareness grows.
- *Listening*  The group members are encouraged to listen to each other. If every participant has a turn in the hot seat, each is the focus of attention for a time.
- *Group development*  The group members get to know more about each other.

## Workers' hints

If your equipment has two separate microphone inputs, use a lapel mike or hand-mike for the interviewee, and a separate hand-mike to pass along the row (page 263).

With a group of eight this game takes some time. You can split the group, and record half the participants one session, and half the next.

Inquiry usually starts at a superficial level. Encourage questions that probe deeper.

## Variations

- Interview several members of the group together.
- Put all the participants in the hot seat. Each person can ask a question to any of the others.

## FUN INTERVIEWS

### Procedure

Divide the group into pairs. One member of the pair asks the questions. The other stands behind them, and provides the arms. From the back they slip their arms through underneath their partner's arms whilst the partner wraps their own arms backwards out of the way.

Each pair interviews one of the other pairs. The questions can be prepared or improvised. The arms use the mike, and provide the gestures. They can point, scratch their partner's head, wipe their brow, and so on. Record the interviews and watch back.

*Average time – 20–30 minutes*

### Value

- *Fun*   These games are a light-hearted introduction to more serious interviewing.
- *Drama*   Participants improvise, responding creatively to their partner. This game can be used to warm up for drama.
- *Production skills*   The group use the camera and practise other production roles.

## Variation

- Partners interview each other using a nonsense language, expressing meaning through intonation, gesture, facial expression and body language.

## SERIOUS INTERVIEWS

## Procedure

After the group members have had some practice, they are ready for more serious interviewing.

The procedure is the same as for earlier interviews, but now more attention is paid to question preparation, shot planning, seating arrangements, sound and lighting.

*Average time – 40 minutes*

## Value

- *Interviewing*   Participants improve their communication skills by deciding what they want to know, preparing appropriate questions and carrying out the interviews.
- *Planning*   Through preparation the group generate video material that explores their chosen topic in an ordered way.
- *Advocacy*   The interview format facilitates representation of the interviewee's views, when recording material for a programme, or as part of the development process.
- *Production*   The group select a suitable shot, and learn more about sound and lighting.

## Workers' hints

Help the interviewer to plan open questions.

Encourage the group to consider the best seating arrangement for the interview. If both interviewer and interviewee are in shot, they should sit quite close for best results. Alternatively, the interviewee can sit in front of the camera face on, with the interviewer at the side of the camera so that the interviewee faces towards the camera when they reply.

Get the participants to work with the available light conditions as much as possible, but it may be appropriate to introduce video lights if recording for a final video.

## Representation

Representation is an important issue when using video. Participatory video aims to facilitate the group's control over the way they are represented, by providing access to a channel of communication through which they can express their point of view to others.

From the very beginning of the project, participants are encouraged to talk about themselves on tape. As the project develops, awareness of how presentation affects the impact of what they say increases. This is facilitated by video's immediate playback capability.

As the project progresses, and the group consider using video to communicate with people outside the group, their ability to get their ideas across effectively is developed. At this stage of the process, the participants' knowledge about how a video message is constructed grows. Games concentrate on investigating the process by which video conveys subtle meaning.

Planning is vital to the group's active control over the way they are perceived. They now also think about the audience they are talking to, how they might be viewed, and the best way to portray themselves. As with television production, a video maker cannot completely control the way in which the viewer interprets their message. The essential point is that the participants are in charge of their own representation, based on a practical understanding of the medium. Their increased awareness of video, combined with a regard for the audience's perspective, boosts their ability to represent themselves effectively.

## NEWS ITEM

## Procedure

Divide the participants into smaller groups. Each group chooses something that has happened to present as a news item. They decide what to say, and how to represent their story. The piece can be recorded in the style of a news interview, or be more discussion-based. It can be dramatized, or related straight to camera.

All the news items are combined in one programme by recording links with a newscaster before and after each group. After watching the programme, discuss how the different styles of presentation affected its impact.

*Average time – 40 minutes*

## Value

- *Representation*   Group members choose a story to tell and decide how to portray it.
- *Ordering of experience*   Participants make sense of their story through relaying it to an audience.
- *Critical awareness*   The group gain a better understanding of the video medium.

## Variations

- *Programme Parodies*   Imitate other programme styles to explore different ways of presenting information, for instance, weather reports or advertisements.

## PERSONAL ADVERTISEMENT

Divide into pairs. Each person scripts a short advertisement for themselves. The advertisement can be themed, covering their attributes for a specific function, for example as a friend, as a group participant, as a parent, or for a particular job.

In addition, everyone decides how to present themselves, including the nature of the shot, and the style of the advertisement. During preparation, partners support each other by suggesting positive qualities to include.

Each advertisement is recorded one after the other, swapping technical roles throughout.

*Average time – 50 minutes*

## Value

- *Self-worth*   Stimulates participants to think of their positive qualities, and encourages them to value themselves.
- *Self-advocacy*   Group members represent themselves on video.
- *Nature of the medium*   The group explore the effect of camera angles and shot sizes, and pick an appropriate style.
- *Planning*   Each member of the group prepares and scripts their presentation.

### Workers' hints

Help the group plan, making sure they consider camera angles and backdrops.
Record 5 seconds of black before and after each advertisement.

## FOR AND AGAINST CHAT SHOW

### Procedure

Divide the participants into two groups. Each group plans two chat shows. Both have the same topic, but in one the interviewer, technical crew and audience support the guest, and in the other they oppose them.

The groups plan camera angles (page 264), question styles and sound techniques, in the first instance to represent the guest positively, and in the second to be as disparaging and unsupportive as possible.

Each group supplies chat show host, camera operator, sound operator and floor manager for their own chat show. The guest is provided by the other group. Record the against chat show followed by the supportive version for one group, and then both versions for the other group.

*Average time – 60 minutes*

### Value

• *Control and representation* This game clearly demonstrates the power of the technical crew to affect representation. Balance and impartiality can be discussed.

### Workers' hints

Use the same guest and host for both chat show versions, to maximize the contrast. Record the supportive show last to end with the more comfortable experience. Get the guest to describe the difference in the way they felt during each show.

Although this game is very effective it should only be played well on in a project, with confident people. Being the guest for the against chat show can be quite undermining, and is not recommended if the group members have low self-esteem.

## MAKING UP VIDEO GAMES

This book covers a wide range of video games to use as part of the participatory process. Many of them were adapted to video for a particular purpose. In the same way you can develop your own video games to achieve specific goals.

Do not be scared of modifying existing games to video. Adaptation often adds an extra dimension and dynamic. For example, Grandparent's Footsteps was first used with a group of deaf people, when developing visually based activities. The results were quite unexpected. The original game is quite competitive, but the video version seemed to encourage the group to work together. In addition, the impact of the nearly motionless recorded footage compared with the group's experience of movement became apparent only on playback.

In deciding which games are suitable for video, consider those that involve some kind of group activity or interaction that can be recorded. Think about how the extra process of videoing and playing back will affect the outcome, in addition to the opportunity for video production practice it provides. Finally, try out your ideas with other colleagues to see what adjustments need to be made so that the game works on video.

# Games index

This index contains all the games and exercises described in Chapters 3, 4 and 5. The main headings correspond to the game categories defined in Chapters 4 and 5. Games from Chapter 3 are also included under these headings.

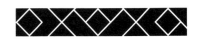

# Chapter 5

# Creating video sequences

Video is an incredibly powerful communication medium because it tells stories, and gets messages across, using the language of moving pictures. Seeing is vital to human perception. People believe what they see more than what they read or hear because of the human eye's function in making sense of the world.

Synchronized sound makes video doubly effective, adding to its immediacy and authenticity. Commentary and other added sound help to determine how the pictures are read.

Video does not show objective reality. Moving images and sound are combined to represent a perspective. To convey meaning in a form that can be clearly understood, video, like any language, has its own grammar (page 265). The grammatical rules define the way in which component shots are ordered in sequence to create coherent messages.

This chapter concentrates on how to work with a group to put shots together on tape. It explains how to introduce video sequences; how to develop the participants' ideas and encourage them to communicate on video; and how to make video programmes.

Remember that different aspects of participatory

115

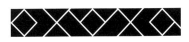

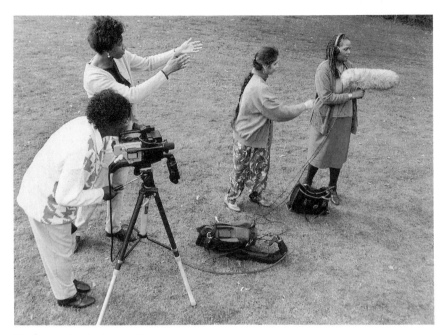

*Figure 5.1* Producing a video sequence

video work develop in parallel through the process. It is not necessary to work through all the games described previously before starting the exercises in this chapter. Most groups put together short video sequences quite early on in a project. The exercises that follow develop the skills needed to communicate with video, and a structure to work with the group away from the workshop space. They provide frameworks that can be used several times through the project with different outcomes depending on the content and context.

## A SHOT SEQUENCE

A shot is the video material recorded between the time the camera is switched on, and the time it is switched off again. Up to this point most games have involved switching on at the start of the activity and off at the end, resulting in one very long shot. This is so that spontaneity is not inhibited while participants get used to expressing themselves on camera. However, the technique of recording one shot after the other is used when several versions of the same game are recorded one after the other, as for the Chat Show; when playing the Disappearing Game; and whenever black is recorded on the tape, before or after a game. From now onwards the focus of the work changes in order to improve the results on tape. Shorter shots are recorded in sequence to explore how to communicate effectively on video.

Video sequences are a basic component of video language. They can be compared to sentences in written communication. Moving pictures are combined in a way that imitates the way the eye views the world. The eye never stares at one thing for very long; instead it darts from one aspect of a scene to another within the field of view. Consequently, lengthy shots on video can be boring to watch because the brain is being asked to fix unnaturally on one image. To maintain attention it is better to record one shot after another in rapid succession to simulate the way the eye flits around. This is why a video programme consists of a mosaic of constantly varying pictures.

Watching a monitor continuously is also unnatural because the eye does not normally gaze at one physical place for very long. This makes video an inherently unstimulating medium. The light from the monitor has to change all the time to keep the eye attracted. If images are edited too slowly it becomes difficult to concentrate, whatever the content.

Cuts from shot to shot are used in preference to pans or zooms. Panning round a still scene with a video camera looks artificial because our eyes do not behave like this. If you look at one side of the room, and then turn to look at something on the other side, your eyes blink as you turn, thus cutting out the pan. It is actually extremely difficult to force eyes to pan without blinking. Zooming is similar. Perception does not zoom. Instead, attention snaps from a wider area to closer up. Zooming with the camera seems slow and ponderous, and often gives a robotic feel. The artificial look produced draws attention to the camera. In fact one of the most obvious marks of a beginner's work is the indiscriminate use of panning and zooming. Good camera work should be unseen, so that the viewer is not distracted.

When the eye looks at a scene the brain does not give equal weight to the whole field of view. It concentrates on one small aspect of it at a time. The brain mentally frames the bird on the roof, the person walking down the road, or the eyes of the person opposite, within the wider panorama. A video monitor already constitutes a small area within the eye's field of view. It is too small for the eye to pick out detail within the picture, so the video maker must use lots of close-ups to define the area of concentration for the brain. This ensures that the feature is big enough to see, and sustains interest. Video therefore works best in close-up, and as such is an intimate medium.

By recording component shots in order to create video sequences, participants learn how to compose a message on video. The results look better, and are of more interest to others.

To run the exercises in this chapter you need to know how to use the equipment to record a number of shots one by one to build up a sequence on tape (page 254). Recording one shot after another takes some practice. Make sure that you are confident with the technique before using it with a group. It is important that you know the following (refer to Chapter 9 for instructions):

- How to set up the equipment in record mode at the right place on the tape.
- How to start and stop recording.
- How to allow for recording time lag.
- How to record one shot after the other on the tape.
- How to use standby mode.
- How to record black on tape.

Remember that if the recorder is de-powered between shots, the recorder can step down and the tape can rewind back into the cassette (page 252). If this happens, the equipment must be reset in record mode at the right place on the tape before the next shot is recorded.

## DEVELOPING IDEAS

Ideas are cultivated through games and exercises already covered, including:

- Statements in a Round
- Objects
- Opinions
- Chat Show
- Questioning and Interview Games

Recording shot sequences provides a more structured way to develop ideas. Participants decide on their opinions, and organize their thoughts more thoroughly. Answers have greater coherence when there is time to consider questions, and the approach leads to measured discussion on tape. Preparing before recording produces succinct communication and aids representation.

### EDITED STATEMENTS

Presents participants' opinions directly and concisely.

## Procedure

Everyone in the group prepares a statement on a particular topic or theme. The camera operator records the first person making their statement to camera. Roles swap round, and the second person is recorded directly after the first on the tape. Swapping continues until all the participants have been recorded one after the other in sequence. The tape is then played back.

*Average time – 30 minutes*

## Value

- *Developing ideas*   Input is generated from all the participants. The exercise can stimulate discussion or develop a new direction.
- *Planning*   The group have time to clarify what they think, and order their ideas before recording. Videoing participants one by one enables them to respond to previous contributions.
- *Production skills*   Swapping provides the opportunity for everyone to practise recording shots in sequence, and learn about soundbites.
- *Representation*   Group members develop their ability to articulate their opinions concisely and to present themselves clearly. The resulting video sequence is a succinct overview of the theme.

## Workers' hints

Record five seconds of black at the start and end of the sequence.

To avoid the Disappearing Game effect, get each person to sit in a position with a different background.

If the exercise is chosen to generate a quick end-product on a theme, set the camera up for a mid-shot of each person face to camera. To be more exploratory, get the participants to choose where they want to stand or sit, and the nature of the shot.

Use a lapel mike for best results, or experiment with a different mike for each shot (pages 259–62).

If the performer starts speaking too soon after the camera is switched on, their first few words are cut off. Get the floor manager to cue the performer, allowing for recording time lag (page 254).

## Variations

The nature of the statements is dependent on the purpose of the exercise, and how the topic is introduced. They can be statements of fact, such as what participants did at the weekend; value judgements, viewpoints or intentions; places to video; or programme ideas.

- *Opinionated Statements*   Pick a contentious topic that participants can express strong views about. Half the group present statements supporting one side of the argument, and the rest the opposing viewpoint. Discuss how participants feel about making statements they disagree with.
- *Progressive Discussion*   The advantage of Edited Statements compared to Statements in a Round is that each person can react to the previous statement, since there is time to assimilate what other people have said. Get every participant to respond to the last person's statement to develop ideas and produce a structured discussion on tape. This is much more engaging to watch than a group discussion.
- *Video Consequences*   Use the same approach to build up a story one sentence at a time. The first person (possibly a worker) starts the story. Each person in the group then adds a sentence, shot by shot. The last person attempts a conclusion.
- *Ten Second Vox Pop*   Record very short reaction statements shot by shot. For example, 'I thought it was great', 'I liked it' and 'I hated it'. Discuss how this technique is used in programme making.
- *Self-advocacy and feedback*   Record all the participants' opinions on a subject, for example the improvements they would like to see in a service, and show the tape to the service providers.

## EDITED QUESTIONS

Produces an edited interview on tape.

## Procedure

The camera operator lines up a mid-shot of a first interviewer facing the camera. Recording starts, they ask a question, and the camera is switched off. The camera operator then sits in front of the camera, and the interviewer operates the camera. The camera starts, the question is answered, and the camera is switched off again. Everyone swaps round, and the procedure is repeated until the entire group have asked or answered a question. Then the tape is rewound and played back.

*Average time – 20 minutes*

## Value

- *Putting shots together*   This game provides a simple mechanism to practise recording shots one by one. The whole group become familiar with the stop–go nature of creating video sequences.
- *Interviewing techniques*   The subject faces the camera directly. This is a common interview set-up, and addressing an unseen viewer emphasizes the concept of the audience.
- *Points of view*   A shot from one perspective is often followed by a shot showing a reaction from a different point of view. This exercise produces interaction between various perspectives.
- *End-product*   Switching the camera off between the question and the answer gives participants time to plan a reply. If the questions are well themed, the end-product is an edited interview, concisely exploring a topic.

## Workers' hints

Asking the question to the camera operator helps the subject face the camera when they speak.

The person answering the question can be confused about why they cannot answer straight away. They may also need reminding of the question. Make sure they are ready with their reply before the camera is cued in.

Reposition the chair for each shot, or use a neutral background (e.g. a blank wall).

Record five seconds of black at the start and end of the exercise to make the end-product neater.

Remember to allow for recording time lag. After the camera starts the performer can count to two or three in their head before speaking, or the floor manager can cue them in.

After the game is played back discuss the technique. The group will be impressed by the difference in pace and interest of the final product compared to recording an interview in real time.

## Variations

- *Question and Answer*   Get the whole group both to ask and answer questions. The first person asks a question only, but everyone else answers the previous question and then asks a new question before the camera is switched off.

121

- *End-product*   Record back and forth between two people or more to produce an edited interview on a theme as part of a programme.

## GAMES USING SHOT SEQUENCES

In addition to the Disappearing Game, other games that can be recorded one shot at a time include: Heads, Hands and Feet; I Spy; Emotions; and In That Way (Chapter 3). The following game tells a story through a sequence of still shots.

### VIDEO COMIC STRIP

Translates story ideas into component scenes.

## Procedure

Divide participants into groups of three or four. Each group devises a simple scenario, for example people stuck in a lift. They represent the story in three frozen scenes: an introduction setting the scene, the middle showing what happens, and the conclusion presenting the outcome.

e.g.
*Shot 1* – People standing in lift.
*Shot 2* – All looking concerned as if lift has stopped between floors.
*Shot 3* – Much later, people sitting in lift waiting for rescue.

Each group's story is recorded one shot after the other, as a series of frozen tableaux, like a photo comic strip.

*Average time – 30 minutes*

## Value

- *Creativity*   Drama skills are developed through devising and presenting a story visually.
- *Group development*   Working imaginatively together in small groups develops social interaction.
- *Programme-making skills*   The game encourages participants to break down their ideas into component parts, giving them a better understanding of drama on video.

## Workers' hints

Video is good at getting across a simple story convincingly. Initially it is hard to stop ideas getting too complicated. Restrict each group to three or four shots, and ensure that the scenario is not too elaborate.

Get the camera operator to tighten the tripod fully so that there is no camera movement. Remind the group to remain absolutely still during recording.

## Variations

- Depict a popular comic strip or famous tale.
- Present a modern myth or old proverb.
- Pick a theme or situation, and three emotions to change through the scenario, for example a party theme, with the emotions of anticipation, shyness and enjoyment.
- Add sound effects; captions between shots, as in old silent movies; or over-dub dialogue or commentary.

## RECORDING SOUND SEPARATELY

The other main technique needed when putting together video sequences is that of audio-dubbing. The audio-dub function enables a new sound-track to be recorded over previously recorded visuals without altering the images (page 256).

To introduce audio-dubbing, visuals created during the Disappearing Game can be used as outlined below.

## POP PROMO

Creates a music video.

## Procedure

Use images from the Disappearing Game. One participant sets the video recorder in audio-dub mode paused on the black tape at the beginning of the visuals. Another pauses an audio-tape recorder at the start of a piece of music, selected by the group or supplied by the workers. Someone else holds the hand-mike between the audio-recorder speakers, and a sound recordist sets the sound levels.

When everything is prepared, the floor manager counts in. They count three–two–one, the audio recorder is started, and when the music can be heard, the video operator starts the audio-dub.

The Disappearing Game images play back on the monitor as the new sound is being recorded. When the black picture at the end of the visuals is playing, the video recorder is paused again. The pop promo is then watched.

*Average time – 20 minutes*

## Value

- *Technical skills*   The group learn how to audio-dub.
- *Team work*   The participants work together to co-ordinate a new recording process.
- *Programme making*   Separate sound is often recorded over pre-recorded visuals when making videos. The group members use the technique to make a simple pop promo.
- *Motivation*   Groups frequently want to repeat the exercise recording a new set of visuals to combine with a particular piece of music.

## Workers' hints

Not all video equipment can audio-dub. Check your equipment, and practise until confident before audio-dubbing with the group (page 256).

Audio-dubbing requires a high degree of co-ordination, and the floor manager's role is crucial. If anything goes wrong, simply set up again and repeat. With some equipment it is possible to audio-dub by taking a lead directly out of the audio recorder into the video equipment. However, it is better, particularly initially, to record from the speakers through a hand-mike. Although the sound is of poorer quality, the process is more obvious to everyone.

Set up sound levels before recording starts by playing the music. Then pause the audio tape at the beginning of the track.

The black recorded at the start and end of the visuals helps the audio-dub set-up, as well as the look of the final product. Initially it provides space in which the music can start and stop. When the group are more proficient the music can be faded in and out over it.

Remember to turn down the monitor sound so that there is no feedback during recording. Remind the group to be quiet whilst dubbing is in progress as any noise near the mike will be picked up.

Do not worry too much about choosing a piece of music to match the timing of the visuals. It is surprising how well a randomly chosen track can fit.

It is illegal to copy most pre-recorded music onto video, without paying a copyright fee. Make your own music, use that of friends or colleagues, or use copyright-free music (page 92).

# EXPLORATION

Exploration is the next stage in the participatory video process. All the exercises covered in this chapter, including those outlined so far, promote exploration and inquiry.

## Exploration of ideas and creative development

Participants are given a framework to examine their experience more systematically. They decide on opinions and organize their ideas creatively on video.

## Technical development

Putting together images and sound to produce video sequences cultivates and explores new technical skills.

## Co-operation

Introducing new technical roles demands greater levels of co-operation, and accomplishing harder tasks increases group cohesion.

## Empowerment

Significant decision-making and planning is involved at this stage. The participants all decide what they want to record and why, and each is in charge for a time. They take greater responsibility for the direction of their work, and self-determination increases.

## Representation

The group gain greater awareness of video production methods and the nature of the medium. They are given new tools to ask questions, and are stimulated to articulate their needs and opinions. Developing their programme-making skills, and providing a channel of communication, increases their ability to convey a message to an audience.

Early participatory video work happens in the security of a controlled environment. Up to this point the project has taken place inside, in a separate room. Now that participants have developed a group identity, and are working together co-operatively, exploration becomes more outward looking.

The techniques can empower the group to venture into the wider world as a unit, providing a reason to leave the project room, and a structure for meaningful outside video production. Participants use the equipment to examine the environment around them, raising their awareness of their situation.

Communication becomes more outgoing through this process. As well as communicating with each other, the group members start to interact with people outside the group through recording and interviewing in other locations. They also explore how to use the medium to communicate their views to other people.

Videoing outside in a range of settings generates new challenges and widens the scope of the development process.


## VIDEOING OUTSIDE

### Equipment

In this context, 'outside' refers to any place away from the project room. Moving around with the equipment, and recording on location, requires a greater degree of co-ordination amongst group members, and new operational procedures. Before working with the group outside the workshop space make sure that you know the following, referring to Chapter 9 for full details:

- The importance of the lens cap (see below).
- How to move the equipment around safely (see below).
- How to wire up the equipment to use on battery.
- How to wire up a portable monitor.
- How to charge batteries.
- How to white balance.
- How to use standby mode to save power.
- How to avoid backlight.
- When to use different microphones.

Working with the equipment outside for the first time is exciting, and the group will be keen to get going. Long lectures at this stage are not appropriate, but it is important that the group understand some basic rules before they start.

## Lens cap

To protect the camera, keep the lens cap on until the camera is positioned safely, and replace it immediately after the shot is recorded (pages 245–6). This is a good habit to encourage the group to adopt even when working inside because the lens cap shields the lens from dust, dirt and greasy fingers. In addition, keeping the lens cap in place until ready discourages the camera operator from fiddling with the camera instead of paying attention.

## Carrying the equipment around safely

Participants must carry the equipment around themselves. They will only take full responsibility for it once they are entrusted with its safety.

Make sure that everyone knows how to lift and carry, and get two people to take anything heavy. Some participants may expect others to carry for them, while others can try to lift far too much. Ensure that everyone pulls their weight, but if anyone is unsure of their ability, or unable to lift, help them. If an individual has real difficulty carrying some of the heavier items, give them something very light, such as a cable or a script.

To save time setting up in each new location the equipment can be left completely or partially wired together. (When using a separate camera and recorder, rather than a camcorder, leave the camera lead plugged in to maintain record mode.) Participants carrying attached pieces of equipment must walk together (Figure 5.2). Emphasize the importance of sticking close to each other, and communicating before stopping or changing direction. If one person stops dead, and the other keeps walking, leads can get badly wrenched. Trailing cables are also easy to trip over so leads must be gathered up and carried carefully.

Make sure that everyone knows which bits of equipment they are responsible for and, on leaving each location, check that nothing is left behind.

## White balance

Going out provides a good opportunity to introduce the white balance to the group (page 245). Explain what it is and get one of the group to white balance in each new location.

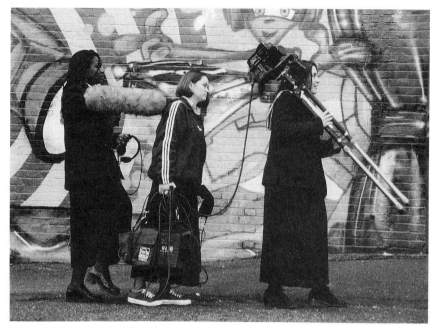

*Figure 5.2* Moving around with the equipment

## Tripod

Continue to use a tripod when working outside. It is almost impossible to hand-hold a lightweight video camera steadily. Any body movement creates shaky camera work, which will dent the participants' confidence, and lightweight tripods are easy enough to manoeuvre. The tripod also increases the security of the camera, and acts as a focus to define a base in each location.

## Operational procedure for outside work

### Preparation

Before leaving the room prepare as follows:

- Wire up the equipment for use on batteries. You need the camera and recorder, or camcorder; batteries; the tripod; the headphones and suitable microphones; white paper for white balancing; and, if available, a portable battery-powered monitor.
- Running back to get a new battery or to replace a faulty lead is time-

consuming. Take spare charged batteries, and any extra leads that might be required.

- Do not forget a video lead for the portable monitor. The audio lead is not so vital because sound can be replayed through the headphones.
- It is quicker to leave the camera attached to the tripod when moving around. The camera operator can carry it by hooking the tripod arm over their shoulder. Detach the camera if it is further to walk, and then replace it on arriving at the location.
- Set up the video recorder in record mode at the right place on the tape.
- Put the equipment in standby mode to save power.

## Moving to the location

Give each participant their first production role before leaving the room. This defines which piece of equipment they are responsible for. Try to occupy everyone by creating enough production roles (page 138), and check that they all have something to carry.

When working outside two workers are essential, as there is more to organize in a less controlled environment. Walk with the group, watching carefully to make sure that leads are not pulled or trailed. One worker should stick with the person carrying the camera at all times.

## Setting up the shot

At each location one worker helps the camera operator to position the camera and set up the shot, in response to the director's specification. The other worker helps the rest of the group to prepare for recording. Make sure that everyone understands what they have to do, and that the presenter has prepared what they are going to say.

The camera and tripod are positioned first to define a base for the location. The rest of the equipment is placed close to the tripod to help protect it from damage. The participants will then need to wire up any equipment that was disconnected.

Take the equipment out of standby mode, and white balance the camera. Ask the monitor operator (page 139) to hold the portable monitor so that the camera operator can see it (Figure 5.3). The camera operator prepares the shot, and the sound recordist sets sound levels. When everyone is ready, the floor manager counts in and the shot is recorded.

Remember, if the equipment steps down, the batteries run out, or the equipment is de-powered for any reason, the recorder must be set up again in record mode at the right place on the tape (page 254). If a shot goes wrong, reset the equipment at the end of the previous shot and re-record.

## Moving to the next location

After successful recording, the equipment is put in standby mode, and the portable monitor switched off to save power. If the next location is some distance away, the equipment can be taken apart for convenience. Everyone swaps production roles and carries the equipment they are now responsible for. After checking that nothing has been left, the group follow the new director to the next location.

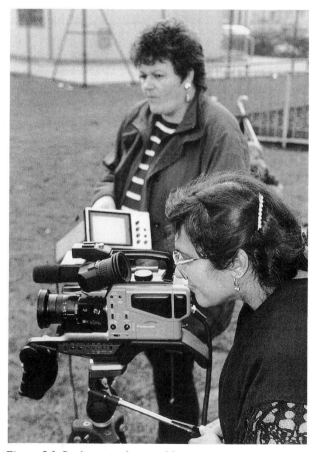

*Figure 5.3* Setting up a shot outside

## THE SHOT-BY-SHOT APPROACH

Shot sequences can be thoroughly mapped out before recording begins, or each shot can be devised one by one. In this latter case the group members choose a shot, and immediately prepare and record it. Only then do they consider what happens next. They then plan and produce the subsequent shot, and this shot-by-shot process continues until the sequence is completed.

The shot-by-shot approach is a useful technique for participatory video work. It introduces programme making through practical experience, enabling video messages to be built up one step at a time.

Participants cannot be expected to think up complete videos until they have had some practice of linking one shot to the next, and some understanding of how a series of shots works together. If they have no idea of how to compose a video sequence, or what the finished piece might look like, it is very hard for them to respond to requests for programme outlines. Ideas will be inappropriate or non-forthcoming, and the group can easily lose heart.

The shot-by-shot approach provides a structured and accessible introduction to video making. Instead of being overfaced with the task of planning a complete video, the group have only to think of one shot at a time. They see how the programme is building up, linking shots by responding to previous action. This aids planning and gives them greater control over the end-product.

When people first start making videos it is difficult to contain enthusiasm, and suggestions can easily get out of hand. Ideas bounce back and forth, and before very long there is an epic feature film to produce in 30 minutes; yet scaling down suggestions always dampens motivation. Working shot by shot avoids this, because the storyline is created step by step. Ideas are contained and plots do not get too intricate.

Communicating in the language of video involves conveying a message through a series of short shots. Video is a close-up medium so one glance can express a great deal. Breaking a scene down into small enough elements is harder than building it up one component at a time. The shot-by-shot approach restricts the meaning to be conveyed in each shot to a manageable amount, and limits the shot length.

Making a programme shot by shot also ensures that planning is not dominated by one or two people. Each participant directs one item, choosing where to go and what to record. The whole group takes part in the decision-making process, and control is shared.

Working shot by shot thus assists the group to communicate effectively on video. The end result is better organized, to the point, technically more proficient, and consequently more interesting to watch.

In addition, recording shot by shot supplies a reason to go outside with the equipment and record in different locations. Instead of videoing randomly, the approach provides a framework for the work. Concentrating on one image at a time also aids the exploration process.

Many of the games from previous chapters can be used outside, but the following shot-by-shot exercise is an ideal introduction to location work.

## SHOT-BY-SHOT DOCUMENTARY

Introduces documentary programme making through experience.

## Procedure

Tell the group that they are going to video outside. Ask them where they want to start. The first person to make a suggestion becomes the director for the first shot. Everyone else is given a role (page 139), and carries the equipment they are responsible for.

The director leads the group to the location, decides on the shot, and outlines what they want the presenter to say. The shot is then recorded.

Ask who wants to decide where to go next. This person becomes the new director, and everyone else swaps production roles. The group move the equipment to the place chosen, and set up the required shot. Then it is recorded directly after the first shot on the tape. The shot-by-shot process continues until all the group members have directed.

Return to the project base, reconnect the equipment to the mains unit and the large monitor, and watch the tape.

*Average time – 45–90 minutes*

## Value

- *Motivation*   Going out with the equipment is exciting in itself. The process responds to everyone's ideas about where to go and what to video so the whole group is actively engaged.
- *Exploration*   The group explore the environment and their situation with the equipment, developing their awareness.
- *Team building*   Group members must interact and co-operate to succeed. Moving round with the equipment, working as a technical crew, co-ordinating recording and swapping roles equitably increases group identity.
- *Decision making and control*   Each individual directs one shot so responsibility is shared. Decision-making skills and self-determination develop.

- *Video production*    Participants learn to put together a sequence of shots on location. Their technical skills increase through experiencing all the production roles.
- *Documentary programme making*    The group make a short documentary piece without pre-planning. The experience means that next time they can prepare with some understanding of what to aim for.
- *Collective achievement*    Participants produce a finished video piece in a short period of time.

## Workers' hints

Each director chooses a shot. Ensure that participants with lots of ideas do not dominate by picking up on their suggestions only when it is their turn to be director. Others in the group can find decision making harder. Simplify the task by asking if they want to walk one way or another, and when they pick a place to stop, get them to choose between two opposite directions to point the camera.

A presenter appears in each shot. This is particularly important at first, otherwise the crew become passive observers of the surroundings. The presenter brings the image alive, and encourages interaction with the environment (Figure 5.4).

It is difficult to complete the exercise during the session if locations are too far apart. You may have to limit the distance travelled between each shot.

If standby holds your equipment in record mode, simply power up, start recording, and each shot follows on from the last on the tape. If standby mode disengages the tape, or if there is no standby mode and the equipment is de-powered to save battery life, the recorder must be reset in the right place on the tape for every shot (page 254).

Ban zooming and panning. This avoids the worst beginners' excesses and teaches the group to put together shots in a less obtrusive manner. In essence, a pan or a zoom is a special effect for getting from one shot to the next. If the director uses a pan or zoom, they are choosing two shots rather than one.

The presenter uses a hand-mike or lapel mike for the best sound.

Record five seconds of black at the start and end of the programme.

To save battery power, do not play back the tape while out on location unless a shot has to be re-recorded or record mode reset.

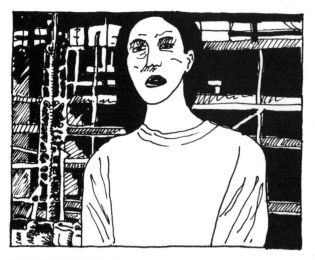

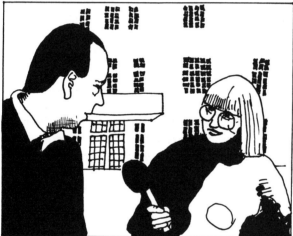

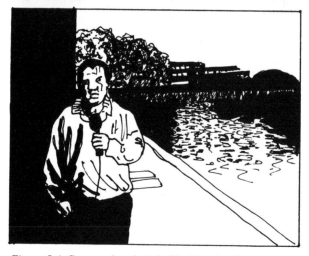

*Figure 5.4* Consecutive shots in Shot-by-shot Documentary

## Variations

- *Looking at the environment*   Produce a shot-by-shot programme about the place where the project is based, for example the venue, the surroundings, the community or the town. Introduce the exercise by saying, 'Today we're going to make a programme about. . . . Where shall we go/What shall we say to start the programme?' Each member of the group thinks of something to show. The last director concludes the programme.
- *Exploring a theme*   Make a shot-by-shot documentary about a particular subject, for example, 'We're going to make a documentary about childcare provision.' Ideas for the theme are generated by brainstorming, or result from interests expressed earlier on in the project.
- *Voice-over*   Get the presenter to speak from behind the camera during recording, instead of appearing in shot.
- *Greater programme structure*   Generate introductory and concluding shots, for example, 'Who has an idea for the introduction to the programme? . . . This is the last shot so how can we conclude the programme?'
- *Increased preparation*   Find out what everyone wants to record before setting out, and plan an order for the shots.
- *Opinions*   When participants first record video pieces shot by shot, they find it easier to describe the surroundings than express opinions. Create a shot-by-shot documentary about a place, or a subject, in which each participant picks a shot showing something that they like or dislike. Alternatively, divide the group into likes and dislikes, and record all the likes followed by all the dislikes.
- *Negative and positive versions*   Pick an issue and record two shot-by-shot programmes, one supporting and one against the subject.
- *Audio-dub commentary*   Record visuals and background sound only, and audio-dub a commentary on returning to base. Try recording several different versions to see how the message changes. For example, record an impartial commentary followed by an opinionated version.
- *Interviews*   Interviews bring shot-by-shot programmes to life. However, restrict the number of questions to about two, otherwise the interview can be longer than all the other shots together, and unbalance the programme.

## OUTSIDE INTERVIEWS

After some initial experience interviewing inside, participants can interview each other, and people outside the group, on location (Figure 5.5).

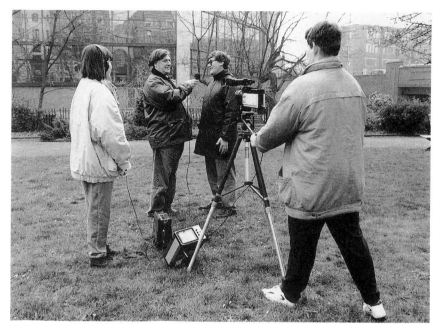

*Figure 5.5* Interviewing on location

## LOCATION INTERVIEWS

The group members interview each other in a variety of settings.

### Value

- *Production skills*  Participants practise recording in different environments.
- *Expression*  Leaving a familiar setting sometimes enables the group to express themselves more openly.

## INTERVIEWING OTHER PEOPLE

Participants prepare and record interviews with people outside the group. Suitable subjects include friends, family, other groups, staff, those in authority and experts on a topic.

## Value

- *Communication*  Interviewing stimulates interaction between the group and other people.
- *Empowerment*  Recording interviews provides the group with a reason to go to new places and to put questions to people they would not generally talk to.
- *Group identity*  Working outside the project venue as a technical crew brings the group together.
- *Production skills*  Moving around with the equipment develops a greater level of skill and co-operation.

## STREET INTERVIEWS

Participants interview members of the public out in the street.

## Value

- *Empowerment*  Street interviews are particularly empowering. Initially the group can feel intimidated by the idea of approaching strangers, yet video legitimates stopping people in the street to ask them questions; in fact many passers-by take part willingly, because being asked their opinions makes them feel valued. Conducting the interviews successfully, and being viewed as a proficient production team, can increase the group's confidence and self-esteem considerably.
- *Positive role models*  It is still unusual to see video crews consisting of women, people with disabilities, older people or Black people. Working in visible areas provides a positive public image.

## Workers' hints

All the outside interviews involve the group moving around with the equipment. Help them to set it up in each new location, in a place that will not cause obstruction. Use a hand-mike outside to cut out background sound.

Make sure that the group have their questions thoroughly prepared before they set out.

Finding people to interview, and explaining to them what the group are doing, is an important part of the process. The group should arrange the interviews themselves. Initially one of the workers can go with them for support. Street interviews are the most nerve-wracking, so get participants to rehearse what they are going to say beforehand.

It takes some time to set up the equipment for an interview. Avoid keeping the interviewee waiting unnecessarily; get the shot ready before finding a subject. This reduces the pressure on the group, and is especially important when working in the street. To focus, get someone to stand in for the interviewee. Mark the place where they stood, and interview at this spot. Set sound levels roughly beforehand, and make sure the equipment is in record mode ready to go.

When the interview is completed, play it back to the interviewee. The small portable monitor is useful for this purpose. Otherwise, let them watch it in the viewfinder and listen on the headphones.

## PRODUCTION ROLES

Video production is essentially a co-operative activity, requiring a co-ordinated crew working technically and creatively together. Good teamwork is crucial to success.

There is a range of roles involved, depending on the nature of the production. In a television studio jobs are highly specialized. There are many people in the chain of production, each responsible for a very small part of the process. Broadcast location drama and high-budget broadcast documentaries can also entail large crews. At the other end of the scale, news crews often consist of only three or four people.

Currently, pressure on budgets, developments in technology, lightweight camcorders and multi-skilled crews are reducing the numbers of people hired. In cable television, camcorder journalists are even working alone both to present and record.

In participatory video work crew size is not determined by the balance between technical quality and budgets. The fact that video is best produced by a team is used to develop co-operation, generating group purpose and a sense of collective achievement. Unlike more conventional video production work, swapping jobs is an essential factor. All the participants contribute to every aspect of the production, and the final result is truly a team effort.

Setting up a shot outside can take some time, and it is important that everyone is kept occupied. Ideally, enough roles are created to engage all the participants in the production process. The number of production roles therefore depends on the size of the group and the number of people appearing in front of the camera.

The list below details a full range of production functions for workers to divide between group members:

- *Director*   Decides on where to video, the nature of the shot and what is said.
- *Camera operator*   Carries the camera or camcorder and tripod. Sets up the shot to the director's specification and switches the camera on and off.
- *VTR operator*   Switches the power to the recorder on and off. If necessary, sets the video recorder in record mode at the right place on the tape. Checks that the tape is going round when the camera is switched on. Carries the recorder if separate.
- *Lighting operator*   White balances the camera and sets up any extra lights.
- *Sound operator*   Transports and connects the microphones and head-phones. Monitors sound on the headphones and adjusts sound levels manually, if possible. Can hold the directional mike during recording.
- *Sound assistant*   Holds the directional mike nearer to the action, or operates a boom, if needed.
- *Floor manager*   Co-ordinates the action in front of the camera and manages the technical crew. Counts in when everyone is ready.
- *Presenter/interviewer*   Uses the hand-mike to present the shot or to interview.
- *Monitor operator*   Carries and wires up the portable monitor. Switches it on and off, and holds it in position for the camera operator and director.
- *Gaffer*   Carries the batteries and replaces them if they run out. If working on mains, plugs in cabling and mains unit. Checks to make sure nothing is left behind.

There are clearly plenty of jobs to keep everyone occupied during recording. In fact there are usually more tasks than people in the group, so certain roles can be combined. Specific combinations depend on the precise situation, but the points listed below are worth bearing in mind.

People often assume that the camera operator is in charge, particularly when a camcorder is used. For this reason it is a good idea to keep the director's role separate. Isolating the decision-making power from the camera operator prevents them from assuming that they are the most important person in the team, and helps the group to value all the roles equally.

It is more appropriate to link the director's role with that of presenter. This makes it more likely that the presenter has something to say about the shot chosen.

Lighting is rarely used in participatory video work, and the white balance can be performed by the camera operator or the gaffer. VTR operation can be combined with the floor manager's, gaffer's or monitor holder's role. A sound assistant is not usually needed.

For a typical crew of eight people the following roles are suggested:

1.  Director
2.  Presenter
3.  Camera operator
4.  Sound operator
5.  VTR operator
6.  Monitor operator
7.  Floor manager
8.  Gaffer/Lighting operator

For a group of four people jobs can be combined as follows:

1.  Director/Presenter
2.  Camera operator/Lighting operator
3.  VTR operator/Sound operator
4.  Floor manager/Monitor operator/Gaffer

Swapping roles every shot is complicated to organize outside. A prepared job-sheet can help.


## OTHER SHOT-BY-SHOT EXERCISES

Like many of the other game frameworks in this book the shot-by-shot documentary is used repeatedly during a project. Each time the group works through it they gain new benefits. A shot-by-shot approach can also be used to introduce drama on video.


### SHOT-BY-SHOT DRAMA

Develops a video drama sequence without pre-planning.


## Procedure

The procedure is similar to the shot-by-shot documentary. Explain that the group are going to make up a story on video. Ask them what happens first, or supply the first shot for them. A shot that generates the potential for something to happen is a good starting-point, for example a close-up of a telephone ringing, a mid-shot of a door opening, or a close-up of feet walking towards the camera. The group records five seconds of black on the tape, followed by this first shot.

Then ask what happens next. The person who makes the suggestion takes over the director's role. Everyone else swaps production roles, and the shot is recorded. A short story is built up shot by shot (Figure 5.6), concluding when everyone has contributed to the story and directed. Five seconds of black is recorded at the end of the programme, and then it is watched.

*Average time – 45–90 minutes*

## Value

- *Exploration*   Dramatic expression, visual communication and the creation of meaning on video are explored. The group learn about video grammar (page 265) and increase their understanding of the medium.
- *Group achievement*   Instead of having one scriptwriter, the story is devised collaboratively, because all the participants choose a shot. The shot size, camera angle and programme composition are more important than acting prowess, so everyone can perform effectively.
- *Drama on video*   Video drama is very different from theatre work. To tell a story visually in an engaging way, many short shots from different viewpoints are combined. With this intimate medium the slightest expression or gesture conveys meaning. Trying to sit down as a group and formulate a video storyline can be difficult and usually produces impossibly complicated plotlines. This exercise produces video drama appropriately, and the result looks much better than simply recording a piece of rehearsed drama.

## Workers' hints

The first time you use this exercise do it indoors so it can be completed in the available time. The plot will be dependent on the environment, the props and the available people.

You may have to be quite directive initially to stop one or two people dominating and to keep the process moving along.

Make the sequence snappy by encouraging participants to pare shot ideas to a minimum. Stick to one piece of action each shot, and restrict the person in shot to one sentence or gesture.

Do not allow panning or zooming (page 133). Make sure you understand editing grammar (page 265). Avoid a jump in continuity by changing camera angle, point of view or location between shots.

Improvise with interpretation on video. For example, a crowd scene can be represented by a few people squashing into a close-up; and fire can be simulated by videoing the scene through a candle flame.

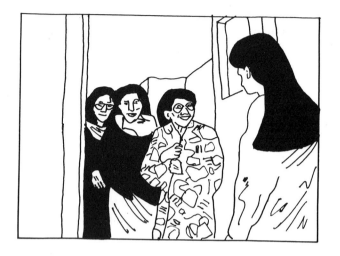

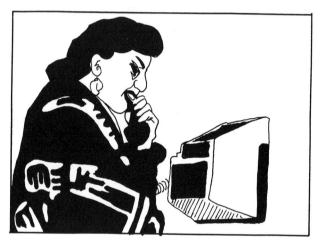

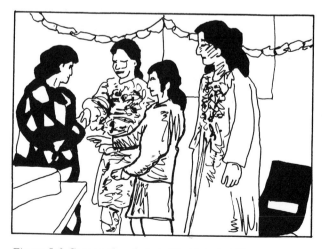

*Figure 5.6* Consecutive shots in Shot-by-shot Drama

Use a directional mike or boundary mike (pages 260–2).

Get the last director to conclude the story or, alternatively, get the group to come up with a conclusion together after everyone has chosen their shot.

## Variations

- *Faces and Hands*   Restrict each shot to a facial expression, or a close-up of hands or feet, to encourage the group to work in close-up.
- *Location drama*   Produce a shot-by-shot drama outside.
- *Represent the real world*   Documenting real events is essentially dramatic reconstruction. Get the group to create a daily activity shot by shot.
- *Audio-dub sound*   Record a sequence of visuals shot by shot, and over-dub sound effects, music or commentary later.

## BALL GAME

Constructs a ball game on tape.

## Procedure

Pick a ball game to represent on video, such as netball, cricket or tennis. Record it shot by shot, each shot consisting of a short specific component of the action. For example, in a netball/basketball version (Figure 5.7):

*Shot 1* – A first player holding the ball, and looking for someone to pass to.
*Shot 2* – A second player calling for the ball, or running into shot.
*Shot 3* – The first player passing the ball, by throwing it past the camera lens.
*Shot 4* – Another player catching the ball as it is thrown past the camera towards them.

The video is thus built up, one shot at a time. Each action is constructed one after another, concentrating on the interaction back and forth between the team players, the opponents and the crowd.

*Average time – 45–90 minutes*

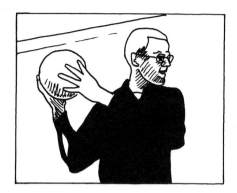

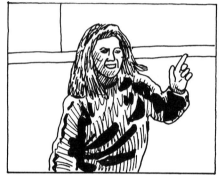

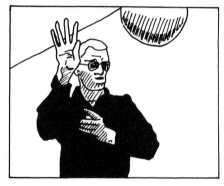

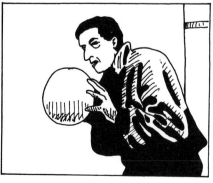

*Figure 5.7* Ball Game

## Value

- *Analysing and ordering*   Participants gain experience of breaking an activity down into component parts, and develop editing skills.
- *Drama production*   Recording the game shot by shot produces a more dramatic result on tape than videoing players actually playing. The simple scenario provides a framework for the group to look at how shots are linked. This exercise involves interaction between a number of people, and the camera takes various points of view.
- *Understanding the medium*   The difference between a real game and creating a game on video questions video's relationship with reality.

## Workers' hints

In the enthusiasm, make certain each participant chooses a shot so that the exercise is not taken over by one or two people.

In general, combine mid-shots and close-ups with one player in each shot.

Make sure that you understand editing grammar (page 265). In particular, watch the direction of action so that the line is not crossed as players run in and out of shot and pass the ball (page 271).

## Variations

- *A fight*   Record a fight shot by shot in a similar way, restricting each shot to one person. For example, in one shot a fighter faces the camera and aims a punch past the lens, in the next their opponent reacts as if hit. This prevents any actual physical contact, and questions the reality of violent films.

## PLANNING

Making shot-by-shot sequences develops the group's understanding of how sound and visuals are combined on tape to create video programmes. Members gain experience of using the language of video and more idea of what is possible in the available time. After some practice recording shot by shot, planning can be introduced.

Initially, verbal planning is sufficient. Participants each describe what they want to video, and the ideas are ordered before setting out. With drama work the general story idea is established before shot-by-shot work on the specifics begins. However, more concrete planning techniques are soon needed.

## Storyboards

Storyboards are visual tools used to plan videos. They consist of a series of television-shaped boxes, each representing a shot. When planning a sequence, a sketch is made in one of the boxes for every shot to show who or what is to be seen in the frame. The image indicates the shot size and nature, and the camera direction and angle. It also signifies any movement either by those in front of the camera or by the camera itself. Next to the box, sound requirements are specified including scripted dialogue; interview questions; and any background sound, music or sound effects. The completed storyboard helps the video maker to assess whether the sequence of shots works visually or not.

Storyboarding is a technique of value in participatory video work (Figure 5.8). Initially it is introduced shot by shot.

## SHOT-BY-SHOT DRAMA STORYBOARD

Introduces drama storyboarding and recording according to a plan.

### Procedure

Each participant draws a picture in turn to build up a drama storyboard shot by shot. A worker can draw the first shot to get the sequence started (e.g. phone ringing or door opening). Then ask the group what happens next. The first person to make a suggestion sketches the next shot.

This process continues until everyone has contributed to the story. Every few drawings, review the storyboard to remind the group of the developing narrative, and establish firmly what the sketches represent.

When the storyboard is complete, the group check continuity to see that the shot sequence does not break the rules of editing grammar (page 265). If necessary, change the shot order or add extra shots to make it work. Then record the drama, swapping production roles throughout (Figure 5.9).

*Average time – 90–120 minutes*

### Value

- *Planning skills*   Participants are given tools to aid abstract visualization and to enable them to order their ideas.
- *Group achievement*   Working shot by shot ensures that the storyboard is produced collectively. Each participant sketches and directs a shot, and the

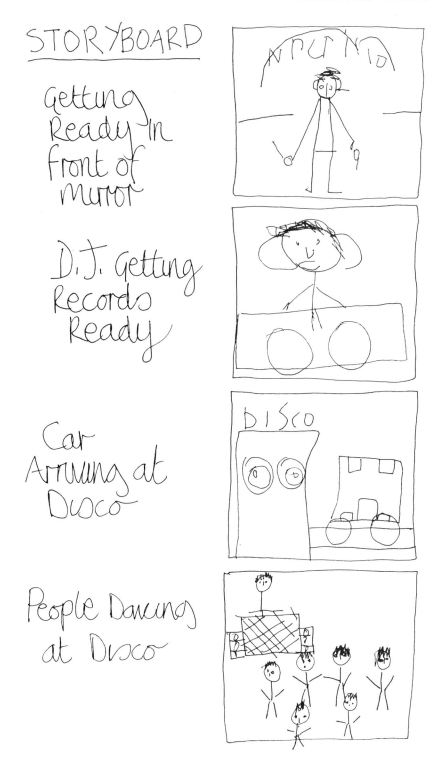

*Figure* 5.8 Disco Video storyboard produced by a group of people with learning disabilities

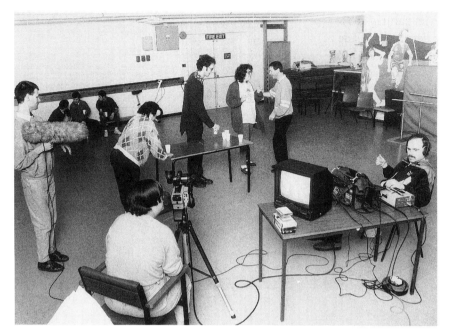

*Figure 5.9* Recording drama

group's responsibility for their own work increases.

- *Editing*   Participants explore creative editing grammar and learn how to link shots appropriately.

## Workers' hints

Storyboards do not need to be works of art. Demonstrate with rough stick figures and discourage competition. It does not matter how well individuals can draw. A squiggle is enough as long as the person who draws it explains what it represents. If anyone finds it impossible to hold a pencil, get them to describe what they want in the picture, and someone else can draw to their specification.

Draw each shot on a separate piece of paper. Shots can then be swapped round or inserted as need be. Also, more than one person can draw at once.

If the sequence does not work, do not cut a shot. This makes whoever drew it feel that their effort was inadequate. Instead, add extra shots or change the sequence round so it works.

The main characters in a drama frequently have to appear in the majority of shots. As they do not get so much production experience, ensure that they have the opportunity to use the camera when not performing.

Get participants to specify any dialogue or sound required in their shot. Note the details at the side of the storyboard.

This exercise takes some time. If necessary the group can storyboard one week and record the next. Make notes so that you remember what all the storyboard pictures represent.

## Variations

- *Storyboard Consequences*   Get everyone to draw a shot at once. Then spread out the pieces of paper and ask the group to put them in order so that they make sense, adding sound as necessary.
- *Magazines*   Instruct the group to cut out magazine pictures, or sentences from a newspaper, and combine them to create a storyboard.
- *Increased planning*   Devise the complete scenario first, and then storyboard it.

## Storyboarding in groups

After some storyboarding experience, participants can plan in smaller groups (Figure 5.10). The workers should keep an eye on the process to make sure that everyone is contributing.

## CAMERA ANGLES GAME

Explores camera angles through a storyboarded drama.

## Procedure

Divide the participants into two groups. Provide each group with a scenario in which a number of characters are interacting, for example a card game or a business meeting. (It is more interesting if they work on different stories.)

Both groups create a storyboard using camera angles and shot sizes to represent the relative importance or power of the characters. There is no dialogue.

Each group then directs and records their drama, using the other group as actors.

*Average time – 60–90 minutes*

149

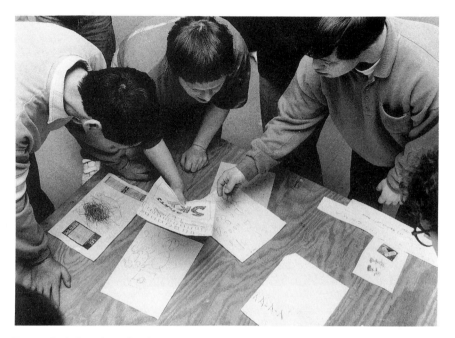

*Figure 5.10* Storyboarding in groups

## Value

- *Group independence*   Working in smaller groups increases participants' self-determination.
- *Camera angles*   People rarely think about the tripod height and set it for convenience only. This game encourages them to consider how camera height affects the image.
- *Editing*   The group explores editing grammar creatively.

## Workers' hints

Restrict each group to four or five shots, or recording will take too long.

Encourage the group to confront stereotypes. Make the tallest person look short, or a shy person powerful. Exaggerate camera angles to emphasize the effect.

Get participants to include facial expressions and discuss how the smallest eye movement or gesture can convey meaning on video.

## Storyboarded documentary

Documentaries can also be storyboarded shot by shot or in smaller groups.

### SHOT-BY-SHOT DOCUMENTARY STORYBOARD

Introduces documentary storyboarding.

#### Procedure

Each participant draws a picture in turn to build up a documentary storyboard. They show who or what is in shot, the nature of the shot, and specify what is said. When everybody has contributed, continuity is checked, and an introduction and conclusion added if necessary.

The group then records the programme from the plan, swapping technical roles for each shot.

*Average time – 90–120 minutes*

### DOCUMENTARY STORYBOARDING IN GROUPS

#### Procedure

Divide participants into two or three groups. Each group creates a documentary storyboard and then records it.

*Average time – 90–120 minutes*

#### Value

- *Representation*  Using storyboards to plan documentaries gives participants the tools to order their opinions and to communicate them persuasively
  on video.
- *Empowerment*  Through progressive development from shot-by-shot planning to planning in groups, participants gradually take greater control over
  the direction of their work.

## Workers' hints

Write production roles for each shot on the back of the storyboard before going out.

## Further planned productions

The exercises in this chapter, both shot-by-shot and planned, provide basic structures for making short video programmes. The degree of planning for the production of a particular programme depends on the group's stage of development. Participants often want to concentrate on drama or documentary depending on their interests, but distinctions become blurred when the group members document their lives. Some further programme ideas include:

* *This Is Your Life*   Create a video piece based on a real event in a participant's life.
* *Record of daily life*   Represent a day in the life of the group.
* *Video diaries*   Plan and produce a video diary.
* *Opinion Advertisement*   Make a 60-second piece communicating a strong opinion about an issue.
* *For and Against documentary*   Produce a negative and positive view of a subject.

## EDITING

Video editing is the process of combining specific sections of video and audio on tape to create a video sequence, composition, message or programme. There are two main types of video editing: in-camera editing and editing after recording by copying from one video recorder to another.

## In-camera editing

In-camera editing involves making videos by recording selected shots directly onto the tape in their final order (page 254). Whole programmes can be produced by videoing the action sequentially, from the start to the end, one shot after the other on the tape. The video sequences produced during the exercises covered so far are in-camera edited. An in-camera edited video can be created shot by shot, or be extensively planned.

The technique is known as in-camera editing because the editing decisions are made before recording, and then the shots are edited directly in the camera to build up the programme. The record button controls the editing process. When it is switched on the shot starts, and when it is paused the shot ends.

## Editing by dubbing

The other major editing technique involves dubbing (copying) specific sections of pre-recorded video material from tape to tape. Shots are selected from the non-chronologically recorded original footage and copied in the required order onto the other tape (the edit master). The original tape is played back on one video recorder (the player), while a second machine (the recorder) records the selected shots onto the master tape. Editing by dubbing can be set up in one of two ways.

### Crash editing

Crash editing involves connecting two domestic video recorders directly, and copying from one machine to the other. Whilst crash editing is adequate for dubbing large chunks of video material, it is unsuitable for accurate editing. As implied by the name, video images are crashed together. The editing process is not electronically matched, and this can cause visual disturbances, such as noise, colour flashing, or picture rolling at the edit point. This is because the video machines are not stabilized, and the control track (page 236) is not synchronized when editing takes place. Some domestic machines have a backspace editing function (page 255) to reduce picture disturbance, but the edit is still rough.

As the machines are not simultaneously controlled, and each edit must be set up manually, the process is also very time-consuming. Even when there is some synchronization between machines, it is hard to be accurate. Editing a programme in this way when edits need to be exact, and can occur every 2 seconds or so, is almost impossible.

### Editing using an edit suite

An edit suite is a collection of video equipment specifically designed for editing, and set up for editing convenience.

The video recorders used are made to editing specification, which means that their recording heads can cope with the demands of continual tape searching and pausing. Tapes can be viewed backwards and forwards, at speeds varying from very fast to slow, or moved one frame at a time. This means that editing points can be located quickly and precisely.

The video recorders are controlled by the edit controller, so that edits are performed accurately and cleanly. The edit controller stores edit decisions for both machines, and performs the edit, synchronizing both machines so that they are stable at the edit point.

The edit suite can also include a vision-mixer, an audio-mixer, captioning, and other facilities depending on its sophistication.

## Off-line and on-line editing

Often one final version of a programme is produced directly. With more time and money rough versions can be made before the final edit, to try out shot sequences and ideas, and to test the programme structure. The 'rough-cut' is referred to as the 'off-line edit' because it is usually made in a more basic edit suite using copies of the original material. The final version is called the on-line edit. It is produced in an edit suite with all the necessary facilities available on-line. With the advent of computer-controlled non-linear editing, off-line editing is increasingly being done on computer.

# Benefits of in-camera editing

In participatory video work programmes are predominantly made by in-camera editing. The technique has many advantages, especially for group work and early participatory productions, compared to editing by tape-to-tape dubbing.

## Access and cost

Even if access to an edit suite is available, it is often prohibitively expensive. In-camera editing does not require any extra resources or equipment, so groups can start making simple video messages immediately.

## Time

Editing in an edit suite is much more time-consuming, and initially less rewarding, than in-camera editing. The same programme takes longer to make, as well as being more expensive. Without immediate visible results the group can easily lose interest.

Later on in the process the participants may be ready to use an edit suite, but it is frequently difficult to find the time needed, particularly with groups from institutionalized settings. Often the worker ends up having to finish the programme, which is obviously of much less benefit to the group.

In-camera editing, by comparison, enables a group to complete a short programme relatively quickly, generating a sense of achievement and the desire to continue.

## Participatory benefits

When recording material to edit in an edit suite, it is hard for the group to imagine what the end-product might look like. With in-camera editing the final product is immediate and tangible, providing constant feedback to the group. This accelerates the participatory process, developing ideas and opinions, increasing planning skills, raising awareness and increasing co-operation. The results on tape are structured from the start, so they look good, and the participants' confidence in their abilities increases.

## Control

Once in an edit suite the additional technical complexity, and the access constraints, often shift control to the workers. Even if one or two members of the group understand what is happening, it is harder to ensure that all participants have equal access to the decision-making process.

Editing in-camera is more accessible to all the group members, and the procedure is clearer. It lends itself to shared responsibility for production decisions and collective working. It is consequently easier for the group to develop and maintain control of their work.

## Understanding the medium

When editing in-camera, participants learn through experience what putting together video sequences involves, rather than having to deal with abstract concepts. They experiment with a range of programme styles, and explore how to create messages and to tell stories using video.

### Effective communication

Beginners often record hours of material. Tape may be relatively inexpensive, but sorting through badly thought-out and mainly useless material is a waste of time. If a group edits in-camera they think about exactly what they want to record from the very start. They soon develop the skills to represent themselves effectively with a minimum of resources. The co-ordination, planning and discipline developed also mean that if they go on to edit in an edit suite they have a more ordered approach to programme making.

## Editing with a group in an edit suite

In-camera editing has its limitations. It is difficult to edit really accurately, and it is almost always impossible to change a shot later without re-recording the whole programme from that point onwards. The shots must be recorded in their final order, which can be inconvenient or unfeasible, and if a mistake is made, the shot must be redone there and then (pages 254–6).

At the start, in-camera editing is an ideal technique to use for participatory programme making. However, if the project is long enough, and the situation suitable, you may want to do some work in an edit suite later on in the process. This can give participants much greater understanding of the medium, and control over the quality of the material produced.

Specific exercises to use with groups in an edit suite are beyond the scope of this book, but consider the hints below when planning the work.

## Workers' hints

Make sure that you understand the editing process, and how to use the equipment in the edit suite, before working with a group.

Recording to edit in an edit suite is different from editing in-camera. In-camera editing involves recording for exactly the same time as the required shot length. When producing footage to edit, at least 10 seconds extra must be recorded at the start of the shot. This is to allow for pre-roll in the edit suite. During editing both video machines pre-roll, rewinding back, and then playing forwards again, so that they are stable and synchronized at the edit point. If the action or speech begins at the same time as recording, the shot is impossible to edit because there is no control track on the tape before the action starts to control the rewind during pre-roll.

When recording to edit, count in, switch on and wait for at least 10 seconds before cueing the action. (Some formats need only 5 seconds, but broadcast-standard edit suites may need 15. Check before production.) It is also useful to record 5 seconds or so extra at the end of the shot for audio-mixing and fading.

Remember that the participants should operate the editing equipment themselves. Make sure that everyone takes turns, and is involved in the decision-making.

In the edit suite it is hard for those not actually pressing buttons to see what is going on. After the initial excitement generated by the technology, watching is quite boring. Additionally, editing by committee is a nightmare. Even a fraction of a second can be the cause of endless discussion. Consequently, it is a good idea to limit the numbers of people editing at any one time. Work with two or three people only, and certainly no more than four.

Do not get carried away by the technology. Edit in an edit suite only if it is appropriate for the group and the aims of the project.

Be realistic about what it is possible to achieve. Even if the edit suite is cost-free, there may not be enough time to edit a complete programme in this way. An average 10-minute programme can involve 100–150 separate edits. With a group this can easily take 25 hours or more, even if it is well organized.

Instead start by recording most of the programme in-camera, and then edit together the in-camera produced sequences in the edit suite.

## MAKING A VIDEO PROGRAMME

During a participatory video project the group creates many video sequences on tape. In-camera editing enables them quickly to produce competent, impressive and persuasive video communications. Whether devised shot by shot, or storyboarded, short programmes are often produced in one or two sessions.

These products are valuable in their own right. The nature of the group, the goals of the project, and the time available may dictate that attempting more complicated pieces is inappropriate. However, some projects may provide the opportunity to work on a video programme over a longer period of time.

### Participatory programmes

Collective video making with groups can take many routes. The specific steps taken in production depend on many factors. Most important is that the workers do not lose sight of the aims of the project. There is often considerable pressure to produce a particular kind of end-product, but making a video programme can be unstimulating if it is not approached appropriately. If the technical requirements of production start to dominate, the group can lose enthusiasm, the workers can take over, and the participatory benefits of the process can be lost (pages 185–6). The particular decisions about how long to spend on the video, how to edit it and what it might involve must consequently be made with reference to the group process.

If you decide to work on a programme, the procedure can be broken down into a number of stages (Figure 5.11).

### Ideas

Ideas for a programme can be explored and developed using a variety of games and exercises including: Statements in a Round, Objects, Opinions, Questions in a Row, Chat Show, Interviews and Shot-by-shot Exercises. They may follow up themes and interests introduced earlier in the project or explore a new direction. This stage should result in a clear statement about the purpose of the video.

A video must be about something, and it should entertain; for a documentary, clarify the message to be communicated, and who it is aimed at; for a drama, decide on the general theme or story.

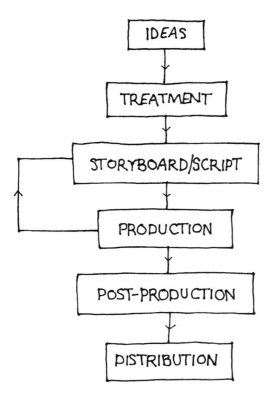

*Figure 5.11* Stages of programme making

## Treatment

At the very start of production a treatment should be prepared. This specifies how the subject is to be treated in the video. The group needs to decide on the style of the programme; the plot for a drama, or the angle for a documentary; the intended audience; and all the programme elements. They choose locations, and characters or people to interview, bearing in mind the length of the video, and the resources and time available.

## Storyboard/script

The group should produce a full storyboard and script before production, including interview questions for a documentary. The quality of the final production lies in good planning. If time is short, it is better to prepare thoroughly and record a shorter video than produce lots of ill-conceived, structureless material.

## Production

Be sensible about the time factor. Remember that editing an entire programme in the edit suite requires a great deal of commitment from the group. Make the first programme in-camera, even if there is unlimited access to an edit suite.

If it is practical to work with the group in an edit suite, start simply. Produce most of the programme in in-camera edited sections, but edit some of it by dubbing. (Interviews are particularly worth cutting in the edit suite because they are difficult to control in-camera.)

It is sensible to edit the whole programme in the edit suite only on a long-term project with a motivated group or if the piece is very short.

## The storyboard/production loop

Storyboarding an entire programme before any production work starts can be over-ambitious. It requires a high level of forward planning and abstract visualization, often without the necessary practical experience, and it can be hard for the group to assess what is realistic.

Instead it is a good idea to work in sections. Choose part of the treatment, and storyboard and record it directly. If the programme is in-camera edited, work in chunks of no more than eight shots at a time at any one location. Then the results can be assessed, the treatment modified and the next section storyboarded and

159

produced. This section-by-section approach allows constant monitoring of the process. The group can revise the treatment according to the results, and the storyboards remain achievable.

## Post-production

If the entire programme is in-camera edited, there is no post-production work to do. If editing is done in an edit suite, the programme is completely assembled from the pre-recorded footage during post-production. If editing is done only partially in an edit suite, the group go on from the production stage to edit interviews; add commentaries, music and other sound; add visual effects and titles; and edit together in-camera produced sections.

## Distribution

This final stage of production is often overlooked. It is, however, vital to a sense of completion and accomplishment within the group.

Distribution can consist of a single celebratory screening to which the group's friends, the funders, people appearing in the video and other relevant parties are invited. The video can also be distributed more widely to other groups and individuals in the area, or via networks on a regional or national level.

# Creating video sequences checklist

*Exploration*

- Use shot sequences to provide a framework for outside video work.
- Explore ideas, the environment and creative communication through putting shots together.
- Encourage communication with those outside the group.
- Develop new technical skills and greater co-operation.
- Experiment with sound and images.
- Make sure all participants make decisions, contribute ideas and direct the action.
- Develop effective communication through producing video sequences and participatory programmes.

*Putting shot sequences together*

- Make sure you know how to in-camera edit.
- Encourage the group to consider video grammar.
- Practise composing messages and telling stories on video.
- Take account of recording time lag.
- Do more planning as the process develops.
- Practise audio-dubbing before using it with a group.

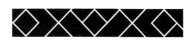

*Videoing outside*

- Keep the lens cap on between shots.
- White balance the camera at each location.
- Charge batteries ready for the session.
- Ensure that the group carry the equipment safely.
- Always use a tripod.
- Create enough production roles for all participants.
- Check that everyone knows which piece of equipment they are responsible for.
- Use two workers.

*The shot-by-shot approach*

- Build up video sequences shot by shot.
- Make sure that everyone directs a shot, and that participants swap production roles.
- Encourage decision making by the group.
- Use presenters in documentaries.
- Discourage panning and zooming.
- Keep drama shots simple, and encourage the use of close-ups.

*Planning*

- Develop the use of storyboards.
- Make sure everyone contributes to the planning process.
- Start storyboarding shot by shot.
- Draw each shot on a separate piece of paper.

*Participatory video production*

- Make sure that the technical requirements of the end-product do not destroy the group process.
- In-camera edit rather than editing in an edit suite for the group's first production.
- Do not be over-ambitious: storyboard and record in manageable chunks.
- Use an edit suite only if appropriate.
- Make sure you understand the edit process and how it affects production.

# Projects

Participatory video can be used with a diverse range of groups in many different settings. It is compatible with those fields of work in which participation, individual growth, communication, group development, self-advocacy or empowerment are goals. As such it can be applied as a tool by social workers, youth and community workers, probation workers, charity and voluntary sector workers, teachers, development educationalists, rural extension workers, health workers, community artists, art therapists, occupational therapists and other group leaders.

This section of the book is about the practicalities of running a participatory video project. It describes how to create, set up and run a project successfully, showing how the practical techniques can be applied.

Chapter 6 places participatory video in the context of other disciplines, considering the kinds of groups that can benefit from a project. It outlines a range of examples to stimulate project ideas.

Chapter 7 explores how to set appropriate goals for a project, and describes how to organize it to avoid problems and maximize benefits. Chapter 8 examines how to plan and run a series of workshops tailored to the project goals.

# Chapter 6

# Applications and project outcomes

This chapter compares the aims of participatory video with other fields of work, demonstrating its application to social work, community development, therapy, participatory education, development work overseas and arts access.

It discusses the relationship between the process the group go through and the end-product, outlining a selection of projects to explore the value of the approach to a wide variety of groups. Finally it explores the issues involved in using video.

## GROUP WORK APPLICATIONS

Participatory video is essentially a technique for working with groups rather than individuals. It is applicable to a range of group-based development work worldwide.

Group work is an approach that brings two or more people together through a common purpose. It assists the development of both the group as a whole and the individuals within it, aiming for change on a personal and a social level. The advantages of working with

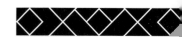

groups have been outlined by Allan Brown (Brown 1986: 13–15) and are summarized below:

- Most social life happens in groups (at home, work and leisure), so they are a suitable environment for work on social skills.
- Bringing together people with similar problems and needs creates the opportunity for mutual support and self-directed problem solving.
- Interaction within the group can change participants' attitudes and behaviour through feedback from other members.
- The group provides a social context in which participants can develop previously unrealized abilities.
- The group can empower the participants. Group members take on supportive and leadership roles, developing self-determination through a transfer of responsibility.
- Groups provide a better setting for people who might find one-to-one work too intense.

Groups are formed for many different reasons, including friendship, support, skill development, service provision and social action. They can be divided into three types according to whether they aim predominantly for change on an individual, a group or a community level.

Participatory video can be used to facilitate development work with these three group types. It generates change on an individual level through developing participation and individual growth; on a group level through encouraging communication, raising critical awareness and building group cohesion; and on a wider social level through generating self-advocacy, self-reliance and empowerment (see Benefits Checklist, pages 190–1).

## SOCIAL GROUP WORK AND COMMUNITY DEVELOPMENT

Social work is an approach to working with people that is practised by workers from many different agencies in the larger field of social welfare. Broad-based social work aims to support people in difficulty and to help them cope with their problems.

Group work is one of the main methods of social work. It is practised by a variety of social work professionals in statutory and voluntary agencies, and takes place in residential homes, day centres, health centres, hospitals, prisons, schools and many other community-based venues.

In social group work people are brought together because they share a common predicament or experience. The approach seeks to help group members to improve their situation by making personal, group, organizational or environmental changes.

It is appropriate to use participatory video with those social work groups that share parallel aims. These include groups set up to generate individual development through increased self-esteem, personal growth and skill development (particularly communicative, creative and planning); those that aim for group development through encouraging shared group experience, mutual support, greater social cohesion and by providing education or training; and those whose purpose is wider social change through promoting mediation, client consultation and environmental, social or political development.

Participatory video is also applicable to community development work. The boundary between this discipline and social group work in the community is not always exact. Generally, community work tackles problems that exist on a wider level within a community, and the purpose is more societal or political. It starts from difficulties affecting a particular section of the community, and works towards changes in social organization, not just additional services. It involves direct work with the people concerned to overcome problems, improve life and generate solidarity. They may develop local facilities, campaign for additional resources, or make their views known. It involves them playing an active role in the development affecting them, and its purpose is that they should transcend and transform their situation, not merely learn to cope with it.

Participatory video is an effective tool for community work because it combines group development and empowerment with access for those concerned to a communication medium by which they can represent themselves. It can be utilized with action groups, pressure groups, representative groups, liaison groups, minority interest groups and other formal and informal organizations within the community.

Participatory video work thus complements a wide range of social and community development work. Projects can be organized with people with physical and learning disabilities; young people; older people; women; Black people; unemployed people; people in care; people recovering from mental ill-health; tenants, travellers and homeless people; refugees; those in prisons or on probation; and a wide range of groups with specific needs.

## ART THERAPY AND CULTURAL DEMOCRACY

Group therapy has a different emphasis from social group work. It is specifically concerned with improving the mental health of the participants through the group process. Its main purpose is to help with psychological problems through improved personal and social functioning. It takes place with children, adolescents and adults who are suffering from emotional distress, both inside and outside hospitals and other institutions.

As well as working with individuals, art therapists use art as a tool for group therapy work. The goal can be to work with particular emotional difficulties on a deep level, but often it is more general. Art therapists work with many groups in the community, not only those suffering from mental ill-health. Like participatory video, art therapy can build confidence, increase creativity, develop personal autonomy, encourage co-operation and communication and realize potential (Liebmann 1986: 8). Participatory video can thus be used by art therapists, and occupational therapists, to supplement and complement this type of work.

There is a fundamental difference, however, between participatory video and the use of video as a feedback tool in therapy. Videoing participants, and encouraging them to analyse and modify their behaviour after watching themselves on tape, can easily be uncomfortable, confrontational and potentially damaging. This use of video is not participatory and needs to be approached with great care and sensitivity.

From a broader arts perspective, participatory video can increase access to the arts for those categories of people who do not typically take part in arts-based activity. This can develop cultural democracy by providing opportunities for creative expression to disadvantaged groups.

## DEVELOPMENT AND EDUCATION

The foundation of education can be defined as the development of human potential. To achieve this objective, education is approached and organized in many ways. At its best, participatory group development, like participatory education, aims to develop latent capacities within people. As participatory video is used to facilitate group development work, it is educational in the widest sense of the term.

One of the major concerns of educators over the last 30 years has been how to facilitate people to take greater control over their lives. (The term educators is used broadly here to include all those who work with people to develop their capabilities, whether in formal educational settings or in more social or community-based contexts.) The resulting methods, from different schools of thought, have been the subject of impassioned debate for many decades.

Lyra Srinivasan (1992: 5) has examined the application of selected educational approaches to development work, defining three strategies currently used to meet perceived needs, as summarized below:

- the didactic approach, which aims to transfer skills and information in order to help people develop new ways of coping with their situation;
- the conscientization approach, which aims to help people transform their situation; and
- the growth-orientated approach, which aims to assist people to transcend their relationship to their situation and its limitations by developing a new perception of themselves and a changed view of the future.

These models can be used to place participatory video in a theoretical context.

The non-participatory, didactic educational strategy is the traditional teaching model whereby the teacher delivers a predetermined content to the students in a formal way. This is the top-down directive method traditionally employed in most schools and places of learning. Paulo Friere has described it as the 'banking' concept of education, where knowledge is withdrawn from the teacher and deposited in the student. Friere suggests that this system actually discourages active enquiry and independent thought. Participants' subservience to the teacher creates a hierarchical relationship that only increases dependency (Friere 1972: 45–6, 57–68). John Dewey criticized this form of education many years before Friere. Dewey maintained that feelings of inadequacy increase when learners silently receive predigested knowledge. Active participation is impossible when content is imposed from above by the teacher without reference to the participants' experience of reality (Dewey 1949: 18–19, 43–8).

The didactic approach is applied in development settings when the 'expert' (worker, educator or outside agency) wants to impart skills or information to help people deal with their problems more effectively. Formal video training courses organized for sections of the community under-represented in the media often use this strategy. Whilst it may be the quickest and most effective method of passing on technical skills in a way that can be controlled, focused, supported and evaluated, it is not participatory. Training concentrates on delivering the required body of information rather than on developing the participants' belief in their own abilities and ideas. A formal video training course using a didactic approach can benefit those people who have already had opportunities to develop their capabilities through education or background. For others the consequence may be to discourage participation, increase dependency and reduce confidence, making them less likely to express their opinions on video (assuming that they are self-assured enough to attend in the first place).

Participatory video practice, by comparison, specifically addresses the needs of people who have not had opportunities to develop their full potential for a range of social reasons. It can be related to the two other educational strategies: conscientization and the growth-orientated approach. They are both participatory techniques but differ from each other in that 'conscientization' aims to generate external change and 'growth' to generate change from within.

The growth-orientated educational strategy concentrates on individual development. As Srinivasan explains, it 'is people-centred rather than issue-focused. It is concerned with the development of *individual* capacities through the group learning process. Its aim is to help people discover their potential and use it' (Srinivasan 1992: 38). Growth in this context is the process by which participants realize an ability to be creative, to have ideas, to make decisions, and to plan and work to achieve a result with others. This process is empowering. Through the project participants discover for themselves their unique resources and inner potential, thus changing their perception of the situation they are in.

Growth is fundamental to development work with people. The participatory video approach aims to create a climate in which individual growth can occur. Participants are provided with experiential group-based tasks, grounded in their experience. These activities allow them to acquire a sense of their abilities. They see themselves as having opinions of value, the capacity to organize ideas and the skills to communicate them to others.

Conscientization is an approach pioneered by Friere and described in *Pedagogy of the Oppressed* (Friere 1972). He developed it through his work teaching illiterate people in Brazil. It concentrates on changing the conditions of society through education by encouraging assertive behaviour by oppressed people. Friere believes that each person, regardless of their powerlessness, has the ability to examine their situation critically in what he calls a dialogical encounter. The educator and the participants, as equals, reflect on and communicate about concerns that are meaningful to the group. This results in an awareness of inherent contradictions and the causes of injustice. The fresh perception of reality, combined with the strength they gain from collective achievement, motivates them to take action to change the conditions of their lives.

Participatory video uses a similar process to conscientization. Participants are encouraged to communicate about their experiences, to use the camera to focus on their world in a new way, and to reflect on their position within it. This mapping process involves the group building up a picture of their environment together. This is the first step towards questioning their situation, and deciding what they want to improve. Video also generates change by providing a means for the group to communicate their needs to those with decision-making power.

These two participatory educational techniques have proponents and critics. The growth-orientated strategy is sometimes thought to lead to individuals becoming egocentric and self-serving, rather than being concerned with the common good. Additionally, in a society where success is supposed to be available to all through personal effort, individuals may blame themselves for failure rather than recognizing societal injustice.

Conscientization is sometimes criticized because stirring up oppressed people to direct confrontation is not always appropriate. It may lead to violence or internal conflict within a community, with little prospect of resolution. Social reform also changes little if there is not a parallel development in people's perception of their capabilities.

Participatory video practice combines elements of the two participatory educational approaches. This avoids potential difficulties by balancing group and individual needs. Individual growth is firmly rooted in the socializing group environment. Participants are encouraged to co-operate rather than compete, and to support each other's development. By combining conscientization with the cultivation of participants' capabilities, the group are stimulated to bring about controlled changes in their environment.

Participatory video thus develops individuals through the group process, as well as the group's awareness, sense of identity and capacity for social action. It is a powerful tool for participatory educational work, and is applicable to development projects in the UK and overseas where it can promote self-directed action amongst disadvantaged groups.

## PROJECT OUTCOMES

In order to define appropriate goals for a participatory video project, an awareness of the range of potential outcomes is needed. Video's suitability for a given situation can then be assessed and realistic aims set.

### Process and product

Video work with groups is often defined as either process or product led, depending on whether the value gained from the group process, or the production of a video, is the most significant factor. This is not a useful distinction in participatory video. Although its primary goal is to maximize the benefits of the process to the group, video material is produced at almost every session. These recognizable end-products may have a small audience and a one-off usage but they still give the project session focus and direction, and creating them is crucial to the success of the process.

It is more important to balance the process and product goals than to prioritize one at the expense of the other. Project planning considers both the process that the group is to go through and the kind of end-product to be produced, and suitable product aims must be set to achieve the required benefits from the process. The outcome of a participatory video project thus has two parts:

- *The result*   The benefit to group members from taking part in the process.
- *The product*   The material recorded on tape at the end of the session or project.

## Different products from different processes

Participatory video project types can be defined by the intended outcome. The games, exercises and end-products suggested in this book provide tools and tasks used to accomplish the established project goals. The project purpose guides the process, and different processes lead to different outcomes: results and products.

Any group video process can produce various products. The project can lead to a tape watched by the group themselves, or by a much wider audience. The low cost of non-broadcast video production means that mass audience appeal is not necessary. In fact one of the major advantages of video as a communication medium is that audiences can be specifically targeted. Video can narrowcast as well as broadcast. The end-product is valuable even if the audience consists of only one or two other people.

In the following examples potential products are categorized by the size of the audience.

### Close-range

The tape is watched by the group as part of the development process, or by one or two people targeted specifically.

### Mid-range

The tape is made to show to a particular local audience, for example the group's community, other similar groups in the area, a particular organization or authority, or other well-defined and limited audiences.

### Long-range

The tape has a wider audience: the whole region, all groups of similar interest nationally, or a mass audience.

## PROJECT EXAMPLES

This section outlines a variety of participatory video projects to illustrate the kind of products that may emerge. Most examples are taken from the authors' work with groups. Others are taken from a list compiled by Iain McLellan (1987: 144), and are referenced.

The examples are intended to stimulate project ideas but they are not the only possibilities. The participants define the agenda in a participatory project so the same exercise produces a different product with each group. The tasks described can be combined in any number of ways, and the outcome is flexible, dependent on the nature of the situation and the time available.

## BRINGING GROUPS TOGETHER

Participatory video provides a catalyst to involve those who would not otherwise meet and increases communication within and between groups. It can also enable people to communicate without meeting face to face.

### Close-range products

#### Interviews in groups

Through asking questions participants find out about each other.

*Example*   A project was set up to bring together women isolated with young children. Using video created a reason for them to share problems and exchange experiences.

#### Street interviews

Contact is made by approaching and questioning others in the street. This is an informal way of involving new people.

*Example*   A Canadian community group, working on issues of poverty, increased participation through video. They interviewed people in the street and then invited them to a tape screening and discussion (Hénaut 1971: 20).

## Interviewing other groups

Video provides a reason to visit people in new places.

*Example*  A group of young women studying to be carers visited older people in an Asian community centre, a hospital and several residential homes. They asked them about the positive aspects of getting older. The completed tape was replayed to all the groups involved.

Mid-range products

## Video letters

In-camera edited statements and shot-by-shot programmes produce direct messages on tape.

*Example*  A group of girls and a group of boys at a youth club worked in two separate groups. They made video letters to each other to exchange viewpoints.

## Magazine video

One programme can combine several short pieces made by different groups.

*Example*  Different groups in a locality made separate video pieces that were edited together on one tape. Producing this magazine-style programme maintained space for each group to work on separate issues, and at the same time generated a sense of belonging to the wider community.

## INFORMATION GATHERING AND CONSULTATION

Video provides a means of consulting those who would not otherwise come forward with their ideas. A range of viewpoints can be collected and information stored for future reference.

## Close-range products

### *Recording for feedback within the group*

Recording discussions, interviews and edited statements are ways of collecting participants' thoughts on a subject. Replay stimulates further discussion.

*Example*   Mothers in a Philippine village recorded interviews about what they fed their family for lunch. This record was watched as a discussion starter on a nutrition project (Atienza 1977: 106).

## Mid-range products

### *Edited statements*

Edited statements can feed into a consultation process.

*Example*   People with disabilities at a day centre produced in-camera edited statements about the changes they would like to see and then showed it to social services planners.

### *Street interviews*

Wider public feedback can be gathered.

*Example*   A rural group interviewed others in the village about their views on local services. The results informed officers in the council.

### *Recording events*

Recording one-off events can inform future planning.

*Example*   A group of Black women made a record of a Black women's conference to promote further discussion.

Long-range products

## Video booths

A video facility set up in a central public place can collect opinions on a subject.

*Example*   A video booth was set up in a town-centre mall. Shoppers recorded their views. The comments were played back in an exhibition about life in the town.

## Planned documentary

A group's viewpoint can be represented through making a documentary.

*Example*   Homeless people were involved in researching, planning and recording a video about the health needs of homeless people. It was used to train staff in doctors' surgeries.

## CELEBRATING ACHIEVEMENTS AND VALUING EXPERIENCE

Self-esteem is boosted by valuing opinions and recognizing achievements.

Close-range products

## Workshop interviews

All participants contribute and everyone's ideas are equally valued.

*Example*   Isolated young people (travellers, homeless people, young people in care and those with disabilities) recorded their achievements.

Mid-range products

## Archiving and documenting events

Videoing events celebrates success.

*Example*  A group of Afro-Caribbean people documented the planning, painting and unveiling of a Black History mural.

## Long-range products

### Oral history

Video is an excellent medium for oral history work.

*Example*  A local history group used participatory video to stimulate memories about their area. They recorded stories and combined them with old photos in a video distributed throughout the town.

## EXPLORATION AND RAISING AWARENESS

Participants explore their ideas and examine the environment. Using participatory video encourages them to ask questions and step outside their normal roles, raising critical awareness.

## Close-range products

### Interviews

*Example*  A group of people with learning disabilities interviewed each other about being called names and bullied. The recorded material was used to further discussion.

### Shot-by-shot documentary

The group build up a picture of their locality together, encouraging them to see their world in a new way.

*Example*  A group of people recovering from mental ill-health at a long-term hospital used video as part of a rehabilitation programme preparing for life in the community. Each week they travelled to a different location and made a shot-by-shot programme.

Participants chose places they had lived and worked in, or that they wanted to move to. Leaving the hospital stimulated them to express thoughts about the past, their life in the hospital and the future.

## Long-range products

### Planned documentary

*Example*  A group of mothers with young children made a programme representing their perspective of life in the community (Figure 6.1). It was later shown in a museum exhibition about the town.

## DEVELOPING GROUP IDENTITY

Participatory video develops a sense of identity amongst people who share a common experience.

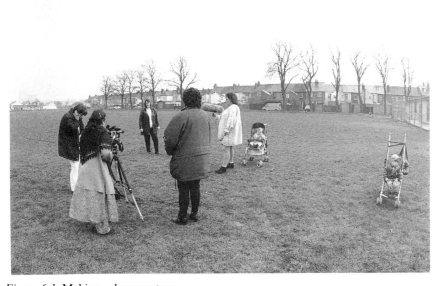

*Figure 6.1* Making a documentary

## Close-range products

### Edited statements

*Example*  A group of unemployed people recorded positive and negative aspects of their lives to compare experiences and find common ground.

### Shot-by-shot drama/documentary

*Example*  A group of deaf people made a shot-by-shot drama about the hearing world. Replay caused a lot of laughter and brought the group together.

## Mid-range products

### Storytelling

*Example*  A group of older Asian people recorded stories to camera to build up a sense of their shared history. It was shown to other groups in the locality.

### Video diaries

*Example*  A group of people with learning disabilities documented aspects of their daily lives. The diaries were shown to key workers to assess future changes, and to other similar groups to generate discussion.

## EXPLORING AN ISSUE

Participatory video encourages people to develop opinions about issues affecting them.

## Close-range products

### Interviews/edited questions

Asking and answering questions are ways of exploring ideas about an issue. Watching and discussing can take the debate further.

*Example*    A group of young Asian women used video to explore their attitude to clothes and the peer group pressure to conform.

## Mid-range products

### Edited statements

*Example*    A group of men at a hostel for ex-offenders recorded statements about life outside prison. It was used as a discussion starter with those just released.

### Opinionated shot-by-shot documentary

Positive and negative shot-by-shot documentaries encourage the group to voice their opinions.

*Example*    A group of Nepalese community workers explored their opinions about environmental issues by making a shot-by-shot documentary representing the positive and negative sides of life in Katmandu.

## Long-range products

### Planned drama/documentary

*Example*    A group of young women identified a common interest in how girls are treated at home compared to boys. They developed a video drama about their shared experiences, interviewed young people on the street, and recorded discussions. They then edited a tape, and showed it as a discussion starter at youth clubs and schools across the region.

## GETTING A MESSAGE ACROSS

Video provides participants with a channel of communication. It puts illiterate and uneducated groups on a more equal footing with those in authority, and they can use it to negotiate without the necessity to meet.

## Mid-range products

### Video interviews/discussions/statements

*Example*   Women vendors in India used video in negotiations with the municipality about their rights to space in the market. Most of the illiterate vendors would not have had the confidence to talk to the government directly. The women's video group recorded a discussion of the issues and played it to the commissioner so that he could hear their problems (Stewart 1988: 15).

### Promotional tape

*Example*   Members of a club for unemployed people made an in-camera edited tape to attract new members.

### Video newsletter

*Example*   Several groups of people with learning disabilities made short video pieces, combined in a video newsletter. As well as developing communication skills amongst the participants, it was distributed to other groups in the area to facilitate the exchange of information.

## Long-range products

### Campaign tape

*Example*   A tenants' group made a video to inform other council tenants about new housing legislation and to stimulate them to form action groups on their own estates.

### Educational tape

*Example*   A group of people with disabilities made a tape about disability awareness for use in training sessions with staff in shops and public facilities.

## CHALLENGING ATTITUDES AND DEVELOPING INDEPENDENCE

Participatory video provides the opportunity for groups to take on new roles, go to new places and challenge expectations. They are encouraged to ask questions, make decisions and take more control.

### Close-range products

### Planned drama/documentary

*Example*    A group of people recovering from mental ill-health made a video about the town they had moved to after leaving long-term institutional care. This assisted their integration into the community, and developed their capacity to make decisions about their new life.

### Interviews/recording in public

*Example*    A group of people with learning difficulties formed their own independent video group. Working competently as a crew in public provided a positive role model and challenged assumptions. They interviewed a television reporter, reversing normal roles, and videoed in places normally inaccessible to them. Taking charge of the project finances gave them greater control over their own work.

## ISSUES IN USING VIDEO

Video as a medium raises a number of issues, some of which are particularly pertinent when setting up projects.

### Participation and non-participation

It is important to be clear about the difference between participatory and non-participatory video work with groups to understand fully the difficulties that can arise.

The main goal of non-participatory video work is to produce a video. Recording planned material of sufficient technical quality is the predominant consideration. In traditional video production, an experienced crew make the programme, with no active participation from the subjects, and editorial control lies with the maker.

In an effort to make their programmes more representative some video producers involve groups in their work. Despite this, the emphasis on the end-product limits genuine participation. In non-participatory production work with groups, participants do not operate the equipment or decide how their ideas are presented. Even in access work, where those represented take part at the planning stage, their input is not based in a practical understanding of the medium. Professionals record and edit the tape and the director has final editorial control.

The question often asked is why should groups produce their own videos when experienced video makers can communicate a message for them more efficiently and more effectively? This misses the point of participatory video. More efficiently and effectively to what end? Regardless of the intention of sympathetic producers to represent people fairly, the technical demands of the medium, and the director's command of the programme, are such that it is impossible for the subjects to have an equal say. All too often they are used as props in the production with no power to challenge the way in which they are represented. Video makers, even those purporting to be community orientated, build reputations as socially-aware producers by manipulating communities to get the material they require. In many cases a tape is made at all costs, regardless of how negative the experience is for the subjects.

By comparison, the point of a participatory video project is to create an environment in which group development can flourish. The purpose is not to communicate a particular message on tape but to establish a working situation through which participants can decide on the issues that are important to them, and gain confidence to speak for themselves. Bringing in outsiders to video the group does not achieve this aim. The group members must actually operate the equipment themselves, whether or not the material recorded is as technically competent. They need to make their own decisions, carry them out, and learn from their mistakes. Only by creating their own work do they gain a sense of their capacities.

It is wrongly assumed that participatory video work takes too long to produce anything worth watching. With a carefully structured approach, an in-camera edited tape communicating a clear concise message to a local audience can be produced relatively quickly. This is more relevant than using experienced video makers to produce to an unnecessarily high technical standard, and certainly less costly.

Even if non-participatory production is the quickest way to make a highly polished video for a wide audience it is not the best way to empower a group to speak for themselves. Handing over expertise to people so that they can produce their own programmes results in more permanent change. Skills are spread, and the development is sustainable in the mid- to long-term because communities are no longer dependent on specialists. This is a bottom-up, interactive and democratic use of video.

# End-product

The nature of the video end-product means that a participatory project can easily become non-participatory. The fact that tapes are produced that then exist independently of the original context frequently confuses the way the work is perceived. Even on participatory projects the product attains importance to a degree that does not occur in, for instance, drama work, where the value of improvization is clearly understood. In drama, any final performance in front of an audience lasts only for the life of the piece and is never watched in isolation from the project itself.

By comparison, the success of a participatory video project is often judged by the end-product, removed from the circumstances that produced it and any real contact with the people involved. Watched out of context, and evaluated without reference to the process, the tape is usually unfairly compared to work made by professionals using better equipment, over a longer timescale, and with considerably more money.

Content and process are difficult to evaluate, so it is no wonder that work is regularly assessed on technicality alone, this being the most visible criterion. However, this results in the project emphasis shifting to the end-product. Workers may then cut corners due to production pressure even when the work is intended to be participatory.

## Expectations

It is hard to get the balance right between the needs of the process and the product. Video's association with television affects what it is assumed to deliver. Most people have watched exciting, glossy, commercial videos such as pop promos, yet there is little understanding of the time and money required to make them.

Funders and managers frequently have unrealistic expectations. No one anticipates that nationally significant tapes will be made by students on an introductory course in video production, but this is expected from groups who by definition have had fewer opportunities. Groups can go on to make professional looking tapes for wider distribution, given more time and increased finance, but a first project, using VHS equipment, is not going to create work that looks like television.

Sometimes the workers' aspirations also put pressures on the project. It can be hard for them to let the group learn from their mistakes, or choose aesthetically displeasing shots, if they feel that their professional standing is judged on the technical standard of the material the group produce.

If the product goals are unreasonable, the demands of the production can start to dominate, and the participatory benefits are easily lost. This can dramatically affect success, irrespective of whether the pressure comes from the funders or the workers.

The group members soon lose interest if they are asked to consider technicalities when they cannot detect the difference in result. The workers can end up taking over and stage-managing the production. The work then bears a strong resemblance to non-participatory production. The workers are simply making a video to their own agenda, using the participants rather than providing opportunities for them.

It is sometimes argued that participants are disappointed with the quality of their work unless the workers intervene behind the scenes to modify the recording. This misunderstands the group's relationship to the product in a participatory video project.

Before they start, familiarity with television may affect their goals, but feedback on replay soon adjusts their aspirations. Technical abilities then grow in parallel with critical development. Initially, group members are fascinated to see themselves on the monitor, and may not notice wobbly camera work. As they become more aware, new technical skills are introduced, so the standard of their work is continually refined. As participants know how much effort has gone into each recording they are proud of their accomplishments, as long as the work is shown in suitable settings and the workers have not oversold the project. On the other hand, if the workers fiddle with the equipment themselves to improve technical quality, the group never acquires a full understanding about their part in recording. They can gain the idea that video production is easier than it really is, and then are more likely to be disappointed if their work is not perfect.

## Quality

Quality should not be judged merely on technical standard. Many expensively produced, highly edited tapes have little to say, whereas a rough-looking, low-budget programme can be very powerful if it gives voice to communities who are not normally heard in the mass media. In fact if democratic channels of communication are opened up, then it is likely that interesting views will be expressed. Much work produced through participation is innovative and captivating precisely because of the quality of its content. The video diaries produced by the BBC Community Unit are a good example of this principle.

They are frequently compulsive viewing despite variable production standards.

Significant work can emerge at any point in the participatory process and its strength is not dependent on technical standard or product form. Even simple recordings can convey forceful messages. Workers can lose sight of this in their desire to make quality tapes. For example, an effective version of Statements in a Round was shown at a screening. Asian tea-pickers handed the mike from person to person and each stated their grievances with their working conditions. The result had originally been shown to the plantation owner in negotiations. Afterwards one worker commented that they would have suggested that the end-product would be stronger if only the three most articulate people spoke. This completely missed the value of the work. An intervention like this could have destroyed the excluded women's confidence at a moment when they were being encouraged to speak up. This was also such an effective tape precisely because ordinary people were representing themselves as a group so simply and directly, without professional grooming.

This does not mean that participatory video workers are content with low technical standards. It is incorrectly asserted that community-based videos are always tedious and incompetent. There is no doubt that there are plenty of videos made by community groups that are hard to watch, in common with many other areas of video production. However, this reflects the workers' lack of competence in facilitating group production more than an innate problem with group-based video work.

Using the participatory approach, participants consider how to put shots together effectively from an early stage. They are encouraged to think about framing, camera work, sound and how they construct messages, and they continually refine their skills. Even if they use domestic format equipment, high standards are expected. The aim is that they produce to the best of their ability according to the project process. There is no reason why videos made in this way cannot stretch the available equipment to its limits and look impressive.

Nonetheless this is a difficult area to get right. It is important to the process that participants produce work that they can be proud of. The workers should help them improve and avoid mistakes. It may well be appropriate to suggest that the camera operator adjusts their shot to enhance framing, or that the sound recordist turns up the mike level if it is too quiet. It can be relevant to interrupt if the equipment is not in record mode so that the group is not disappointed when nothing is recorded. However, there is always a fine line between this kind of intervention and that where the workers prevent the group from learning by fixing everything for them. It very much depends on the stage of the work, the individuals in the group and the purpose of the exercise. The workers must continually weigh up the needs of process compared to the product, and deciding on whether to intervene is often a question of the intention behind the intervention, and the attitude of the workers to the process they are engaged in.

### Appropriateness

The benefits of the group video process are highest when identifiable products are produced, but it is not necessary to attempt an epic, and working on an over-ambitious tape before the group is ready destroys participation. It is obvious that the intended product must be appropriate to the overall purpose of the work. For instance, if the aim is to encourage people with learning difficulties to communicate their needs to social services, it is a waste of time to spend six months planning, recording and editing a tape to broadcast standard. As well as being more costly, it is also likely to be less valuable. Whatever the group members say is likely to be out of date by the time the tape is finished, and anyway, if participants have not developed an awareness of their needs, or the ability to communicate them to others, they are unlikely to say much in front of a broadcast camera and lights. It is more relevant to use video to develop their understanding of their needs, and then to produce a shot-by-shot sequence that expresses what they want simply and quickly.

The context in which the tape is viewed is pivotal. The audience will not notice the technical standard if the content has a resonance with them. Broadly speaking, close- or mid-range products watched by people who know the subjects do not need to be as highly polished as products intended for strangers.

In order to encourage professional participatory work it is crucial that projects are evaluated appropriately, and the end-product should not be considered in isolation from the project.

## Control

A video project is only truly participatory when the control of the project direction is transferred to the participants. Whilst the workers choose the exercises and set the tasks, the specific content is defined by the group. If the theme or form of the end-product is pre-defined by the workers, or the funders, before the project starts, the participants can never develop full control over their own agenda. Motivation is likely to decrease, and involvement will be hard to maintain because the group's opportunity to define the issues that are important to them no longer exists.

Even if it is not explicitly stated, funders commonly want a video produced about an issue that they have chosen for the group. For instance, people with disabilities are expected to make programmes about access, or young people about youth provision. Another familiar variation on this situation occurs when managers see the video group as a cheap way to get a promotional video made. These attitudes marginalize the group. They are given access to a communication medium but only on someone else's terms. Obviously the group's experiences will affect their perspective but they may want to address education, make a thriller, try video art, or create their own soap.

Workers must avoid setting up projects with a limited agenda or themes that are rigidly fixed. In particular, be warned about situations where the group has decided what they want to do before the project starts, with no practical experience of what is possible. This only results in disappointment if their ideas are impractical, and more often than not the idea has been planted by someone with influence over them. If this is the case they will quickly lose interest when work begins. If the subject is to be clearly grounded in the participants' interests, it should be developed as part of the project.

Of course, video workers also have the power to affect the group's decisions. However, they should use their influence to expand the participants' understanding of the medium and develop real choices. It is useful to see the workers' relationship with the group as a partnership, to which the group members bring their ideas, enthusiasm and potential, and the workers bring their knowledge of video and group work skills. The outcome is a result of this partnership.

# Benefits checklist

The benefits of participatory video can be summarized as follows:

*Individual purpose*

Participation

- Motivation and active involvement.
- Response to participants' experience and interests.
- Generation of participants' input into process.

Individual development

- Creativity and experimentation.
- Confidence and self-esteem.
- Expression of feelings and opinions.
- Reflection, self-awareness and self-definition.
- Self-validation and self-belief.
- Technical and social skills.
- Personal achievement.
- Realization of potential.

*Group purpose*

Communication

- Interaction.
- Sharing experience and information.
- Listening.
- Discussion.
- Questioning.

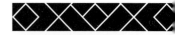

## Community building

- Trust, understanding, mutual support and co-operation.
- Group identity and social cohesion.
- Collective strength and achievement.

### *Critical awareness and consciousness raising*

- Focusing attention.
- Exploring environment.
- Questioning situation.
- Critical understanding.
- Changed perception.
- Development of ideas and issues.

### *Community purpose*

## Self-advocacy

- Development and organization of opinions.
- Articulation of needs.
- Representation using communication medium.
- Creation of new voices.

## Capacity development and self-reliance

- Cultivation of abilities and potential.
- Decision making and planning.
- Problem solving.
- Self-realization and self-reliance.
- Control and responsibility.
- Self-direction and self-determination.

## Empowerment

- Taking action.
- Gaining organizational and political strength.
- Participation in decision making.
- Influencing power structures.
- Bringing about change.

# Chapter 7

# Setting up a project

The success of a participatory video project is fundamentally determined by how it is set up. Groundwork undertaken before a project begins may lack the excitement of the face-to-face work but it is vitally important. It requires as much attention as the project sessions themselves. Many of the potential problems can be avoided by forethought and careful preparation.

The need for consultation, partnership, accountability, participant involvement and effective monitoring is common to all participatory projects. Using video creates additional organizational demands that must also be considered.

This chapter explains how to set up a video project so that it fulfils its aims successfully. Project creation, project aims, project structure, project organization, project management and administration are all examined.

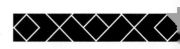

## PROJECT CREATION

### Why video?

Video projects are initiated in a number of ways. The idea for a video project may be yours, a colleague's, or come from a group themselves. The project can arise from previous work or seem the best method to fulfil a specific aim or engage with a particular issue.

Before setting up a project it is important to consider whether video is the most suitable medium for the situation. Frequently the temptation is to use it simply because of its novelty or its availability.

Video is relatively expensive, it needs multi-skilled workers, it can break down, and it requires an electricity supply (if only to charge batteries). Critics argue that drama, song, dance, other media or even group discussions can lead to the same results more quickly and cheaply. However, as previously discussed, video has some very specific benefits. It can motivate those who might be put off by more traditional tools. It can respond to local oral traditions, and is a powerful communication medium for those who cannot read or write. It is highly accessible, easy to transport and anyone can operate it; and its immediate feedback capability provides the group with a new way to participate in evaluation, planning and decision making.

Participatory video is actually relatively low cost when the potential value is taken into account, especially if equipment is borrowed or hired rather than bought.

### Setting up a project

Details of the setting-up process vary with each project but the basic principles are the same. All the elements of the project must be considered at the planning stage. A problem identified in advance is more easily solved than one that comes to light only during the project. Once any potential obstacles have been recognized, a strategy to deal with them can be developed.

Setting up is dominated by negotiation and consultation. If no formal structure exists, it is useful to form a group that can support the project's development. Discussions, either in meetings or informally, provide an opportunity to explore the working environment, what the project can achieve, and its limitations.

Special care must be taken to ensure maximum participation by potential group members in the decision-making process. This gives them a sense of project ownership right from the start. Members of staff, centre users and other interested parties are also more likely to be supportive of the work if their opinions are valued.

There are several stages involved in setting up a participatory video project, as outlined below.

## Creating the project

Includes developing the original idea, research and consultation, assessing project viability and agreeing the aims.

## Deciding on the project structure

Involves making decisions about membership of the group, number and frequency of sessions, workers, administration, management, monitoring and evaluation.

## Organizing the project

Entails arranging the venue, equipment and other resources.

## Finalizing the proposal

Involves preparing and agreeing the budget and timetable, and identifying funding.

# The project co-ordinator's role

Video projects require considerable organization. Identifying someone to take responsibility for project co-ordination can help to ensure effective consultation, planning and management.

The co-ordinator can be a staff member wanting to run a video project with their usual group, a manager arranging a video project for others to work on, or a sessional worker coming in from outside. The responsibilities can be undertaken by a team, but usually one person co-ordinates and administers the work.

The co-ordinator initiates debate about the project and manages the planning process. If one person is responsible for all the work it is important that they are clear about the various roles involved, especially if they also intend to run the sessions.

One of the first tasks is to discuss the project informally with all the interested parties. More formal meetings follow which need to be focused and productive. If negotiations go on for too long the impetus can be lost. Keep everyone fully informed about how preparations are going, and record and circulate any decisions made in order to minimize misunderstanding.

People are often unaware of the potential video offers, or they can have unrealistic expectations about what a project can deliver. It may be necessary to spend time convincing others of the value of participatory video, so it is essential that you are clear about what you want to achieve and the approach you are employing.

Do not be afraid to seek advice, although remember that people with video production knowledge do not necessarily know how to work with groups. Go to them for technical advice, but talk to an experienced group worker about the project structure and content.

## Project perspectives

Who is consulted naturally varies from project to project. Centre workers and managers, other agency professionals, teachers, key workers, community workers, video workers, funders, parents and, of course, the participants themselves can all be involved. Generally a different emphasis is placed on the work by people depending on their perspective. Allan Brown identifies three positions taken with respect to group work (Brown 1986: 28):

- The agency perspective
- The practice perspective
- The client perspective

For example, managers and staff at day centres, schools or hospitals will place the project within the wider work of their organization or agency. Video workers are likely to approach the project from the practice perspective, looking at how the participatory process will take place. The clients themselves, of course, have their own varied reasons for wanting to take part.

A video project was suggested at a day centre for people with learning disabilities. The centre management saw the project as an opportunity for staff to collect feedback on personal development and to develop social skills. Project workers at the centre felt that video was an ideal tool to use with the group to explore issues, travel out of the centre and meet new people. The participants wanted to appear on video and liked the idea of going out of the centre to record.

There were initially a number of potential conflicts. The managers did not fully grasp the participatory nature of the project, and saw video merely as an analytical recording medium. The workers were placing too much emphasis on issue-based work before the group were really ready for it. The participants had not yet used the equipment and needed time to appreciate what video work involved and the commitment required on a longer-term project. Discussions allowed differences to be resolved before the project started.

To reach agreement on the aims and structure of a project it is therefore essential to take account of all the various outlooks. Everyone concerned must fully understand and support the project goals.

## Consulting participants

The participants should be consulted to ensure project accountability, yet this is not a straightforward issue. Their needs may emerge fully as part of the development process only after the workshop sessions have begun. If they are consulted before the project starts, they can lack the confidence to express themselves, and they may not be equipped to make informed choices.

A taster session, some time in advance of the project proper, provides an opportunity for the group to find out at first hand what video is like. Possible issues can be introduced in a meaningful way, and participants can then make a decision about whether to take part in a longer project based on their experience. This also provides an early opportunity for them to input their opinions.

## PROJECT AIMS

The aims provide the basis for the project and should be agreed only after thorough discussion. They should be specific to the group and to the project environment.

The procedure for setting aims can be divided into the following stages:

- Consider situation and needs.
- Prioritize benefits required from video project.
- Identify group and propose project structure.
- Think through possible outcomes.
- Recheck suitability of video.
- Propose aims.
- Decide if aims are achievable.
- Refine and agree aims.

## Consider situation and needs

You may already be running a group with whom you want to use video. Alternatively you may be in a working environment or situation with needs that you think video could help fulfil. The circumstances in which the project is to be run will inform the project planning.

A participatory video project run with a group of older people illustrates how to establish aims. The setting was a large, new estate built primarily for young professionals buying their own homes, but with an increasing older population. Many couples had brought a parent to the estate with them, who then remained when they moved on. Substantial numbers of older people now lived there, uprooted from their previous lives and friends, and isolated in an area with few facilities and little public transport.

## Prioritize benefits

A project is more likely to succeed if it is well focused. Examine the possible benefits of participatory video, then make a list, in order of priority, of three or four specific benefits you want the project to achieve.

Video was felt to offer benefits to older people on the estate through its potential to:

- Improve contact and communication.
- Promote active participation.
- Develop a shared identity amongst isolated older people on the estate, and sense of belonging to their new community.
- Highlight problems faced by older people, by providing a means for them to express their needs.

## Identify group and propose project structure

Next identify the group and work out the time, money and resources available for the project.

A group of older people attending a lunch club at the community centre were identified and approached to become project participants. A twenty-session project with weekly sessions was proposed. The project was arranged on a different day to the club to ensure that it had a separate identity, and so that it did not interfere with other activities.

## Think through possible outcomes

Explore all the various directions the project could take, and the possible outcomes, given the timescale and situation. Be realistic to avoid setting impossible targets both in terms of the result of group development work and the end-products on tape.

While the video project was being set up the group talked to other older residents. This research emphasized the need to contact other isolated people through the project and suggested using the recorded material (whether workshop material or a final video) to promote discussion about older people's needs on the estate.

## Recheck suitability of video

After a taster session or an introductory series of workshops it is wise to reconsider video's suitability. If equipment is readily available there may be a strong temptation to continue working with it. Remember, a lot of the reasons why video appeals initially to groups may not be sustainable over a longer-term project. Reflect on all the available information before proceeding with the project.

Taster sessions with the lunch club helped to clarify what video involved, and to reassure those that were less confident about video that they could use it. They were already quite enthusiastic about the project, but they were even more attracted to video once they fully understood that they would be active in operating the equipment themselves.

## Propose aims

Aims should be specific and to the point, so write them down succinctly. If they are too general, it will be impossible to evaluate whether they have been accomplished. They should be appropriate to the needs of the group, and achievable given the time and resources available.

The aims for the older people's video project were:

- To encourage group members to communicate with each other and to bring together other older people in the community by approaching and interviewing them on location.
- To involve older people actively in the issues affecting them. To promote positive images of the capabilities of older people through their competent use of video equipment and their participation in the community.
- To record older people's memories, feelings and attitudes in order to value their experience and achievements and help them develop an older people's culture in the area.
- To produce video material to use in promoting discussion with council service-providers about the problems faced by older people and the facilities required.

## Decide if aims are achievable

The aims should be reexamined with reference to the project situation to ensure that they are appropriate.

The core group was stable, enthusiastic and committed to the work. Video workers and local community workers were available to support them.

## Refine aims

Finally, aims should be refined and agreed as the basis for the project.

Group participants, community workers and video workers drew up and agreed a proposal. This was used to raise funds and the project duly went ahead.

## PROJECT STRUCTURE

Once the aims are agreed, more detailed planning about the project structure can take place. Matters relating to the group, the workers, the timescale, the venue and the resources must all be considered.

## The group

### Group size

Video sessions work best with relatively small groups. If the group is too large, participants can be under-stimulated and lose interest. On the other hand, if it is too small, there can be too few people to perform all the tasks or break into sub-groups. In most situations five to eight participants is ideal. This is large enough to generate creativity but at the same time allows reasonable access to the equipment and the workers' time.

There is often considerable pressure, financial and organizational, to work with large groups. Institutions, such as schools, frequently find it difficult to timetable for small groups. In addition, big groups are seen as a safety mechanism in case people stop coming. Resist pressure to swell numbers. If participants are fully absorbed in the work, they are far less likely to drop out.

If there is a lot of interest in the project, run more sessions to accommodate numbers, even if they have to be shorter. Participants benefit far more from a one-hour workshop with eight people than two hours with 16. A project can be enlarged to include more people by running several groups in parallel.

### Open or closed groups

Closed groups, in which the membership is fixed throughout the project, have clear advantages for group development compared to open groups, where members can come and go. Introducing new people after the first session is very disruptive, and if the group changes regularly it is impossible to progress beyond introductory exercises.

The project environment often determines whether groups are open or closed. At a hectic drop-in centre it may be impossible to run a closed group, but there are benefits from involving as many people as possible over a number of weeks. Running a series of sessions open to anyone also provides the opportunity for participants to decide if they want to join a longer project in a closed group.

## Group selection

Participants are recruited to video projects in a number of ways:

- An existing group may choose to undertake a video project. In this case selection is an issue for the group itself.
- The group is self-selected. Participants opt to take part, for instance by

coming to a project advertised in their locality or centre. This requires considerable motivation and self-assurance on their part.

• Identified individuals or groups are approached by workers or agencies. For example, a community worker targets unemployed people in the area for a project.

People should always have a choice about whether they join a project or not. However, some may need encouragement, and others may not want to commit themselves unless they know what they are required to do. A taster session can help people decide if they want to be involved (page 196).

It is often necessary to identify particular sectors of the wider community to target in order to ensure that opportunities are created for a range of people, and not just those confident enough to attend unprompted. Consult with the relevant communities when considering how to recruit participants.

## Group composition

The goals of a participatory project are normally defined in relation to the make-up of the group. The group's composition can be defined by the participants' descriptive attributes (for instance, they may be aged 11–14, men, or Afro-Caribbean) or it can be defined by their circumstances or experience (for instance, they may be single parents, patients, or centre-users).

Groups work best when participants are at ease with each other. This creates a comfortable environment in which to examine issues, where all members can participate equally and where no one is disadvantaged by the other members' attitudes. Redl's law of 'optimum distance' states that 'groups should be homogeneous enough to ensure stability and heterogeneous enough to ensure vitality' (Redl 1951; see Brown 1986: 37).

Factors such as the participants' gender, age, skill level and language should be considered when setting up the project. Individuals can inadvertently be placed in a difficult position if they are in a minority. Avoid creating a situation where a single person is isolated within a group.

### Single experience

Groups in which there is a single identifiable experience shared by all the participants provide a supportive structure for participatory video work. For instance, single-sex groups are relevant not only when dealing with gender-based issues or in anti-sexist work. In mixed groups, women are often undermined when learning how to use technical equipment, and so women-only projects allow women to gain confidence using video in an environment where they feel less judged.

It is also better if the age range within the group is not too large. This is especially true when working with young people, where two or three years represents a significant gap.

Problems can be caused by single-experience work in mixed environments. If people feel excluded, they can disrupt the work. For instance, a young women's video group was set up on a separate night from the youth club to avoid continual interruptions.

## Issue-based work

Single-experience groups are susceptible to pressure to produce work on specific issues. Ex-psychiatric patients do not necessarily want to discuss mental health, and people with disabilities have opinions on a range of issues, not just disability (page 188).

If the project is to be issue-based, think carefully about the group's composition, particularly if the subject is emotive or sensitive. Do not place anyone in a position where they are expected to provide answers for the rest of the group, or defend an isolated position because other members of the group feel threatened. This is embarrassing and undermining for the individual concerned and damaging to the developmental process.

## Mixed-experience groups

Single-experience groups can reinforce a sense of difference, when what many marginalized people want is to feel part of the mainstream society. Participants should have sufficient shared experience to make the group workable, but there are situations and projects that specifically call for groups of mixed experience. There are benefits to be gained from bringing together people who might not otherwise meet, to improve integration or to build confidence in a new environment (page 204).

# Project workers

The workers are obviously an important element in any project, and there are many factors to consider when choosing them:

- Do they have the skills and experience to run the project, and do they support the approach?
- Are they available at the times required, and are they committed enough to complete the project? It can be disturbing for the group to have to change workers mid-project.
- Can they develop a good working relationship with the group and other people in the situation? The success of a project can often depend on the help and support of other members of staff.
- Do the workers have local knowledge, and are they required for follow-up work after the project has finished? Even if they are relatively inexperienced, local workers with a commitment to the group may, with support and training, offer a better long-term option than highly experienced workers who have to travel miles, do not know the area and are unlikely to want to continue beyond the project's term.
- Are the workers appropriate for the group? Providing workers who share the group's experience, such as Black workers to work with Black people, is important, particularly for issue-based work and in order to provide role models. However, workers from under-represented groups often become marginalized because they are employed only on certain projects. Workers representing sections of society who are not generally seen using technical equipment, such as people with disabilities, should be considered for work with all groups.
- Do the workers know the group? Workers may already have an established relationship with the group. Familiar faces can make it easier for the participants to relax. The workers understand individual needs right from the start, and may have specialist skills required for the project, such as sign language. They must be on their guard, however, about making too many assumptions about the project direction or what the group can achieve. Workers from outside the environment are often seen as experts and their opinions can carry more weight. This can make it easier for them to introduce new ideas, but they will not necessarily know all the ins and outs of the situation. A combination of a worker who knows the group and one coming from outside can be very effective.

## Timescale

The frequency and duration of workshop sessions varies according to the situation. Weekly sessions are typical; if held less often, the impetus may be lost. Conversely, if sessions are too frequent, particularly at the beginning, the group can feel overwhelmed. Later on more intensive work may be called for, and sessions can be more frequent.

It is common to start with shorter sessions (one to one and a half hours) and extend their length as the project develops (page 215). The length of project elements can also increase as the project progresses. Start with a one-off taster session, followed by a five- or ten-session introduction. If the group wants to carry on then a major project may be called for.

Make sure that the time of the workshop is convenient for the participants, and avoid varying the time, place or day of a session, as this can lead to confusion. Nevertheless most projects do require some flexibility in timetabling, especially if the group wants to record an event or interview a busy person.

## PROJECT ORGANIZATION

It is essential that the project environment and resources are organized in advance. Rectifying difficulties caused by inappropriate venues and inadequate resources once the project has begun can be very disruptive.

### Venue

Always visit the venue before the project to ensure its suitability. It must be comfortable, neutral, physically accessible, unintimidating and safe. Ideally there should be somewhere warm and dry for participants to wait before the session and a place to get refreshments. The venue also needs suitable surroundings in which the group can video safely when they first work outside.

An accessible ground-floor space is more convenient for everyone. Stairs can present difficulties not only for people with limited mobility and those in wheelchairs but also for able-bodied people carrying equipment or pushchairs. Accessible toilets are also required.

The type of venue also has an effect on the project's development. Schools, church halls, art centres, hospitals and many other environments have emotional associations for people. Discuss possible sites with the group; better alternatives may be suggested. Sometimes various venues are utilized during the project. For instance, it can start in a familiar setting to build confidence, before moving to a more challenging location.

Finally, make sure that staff on site know about the project. Their assistance may be required if problems arise.

## The workshop space

The room in which the workshop takes place has to meet certain physical criteria as well as providing suitable conditions in which to work. It should be quiet, private, the right size, and have natural light and an electricity supply.

The room must provide ample space for the equipment and chairs and be big enough for the participants and workers to move about easily and safely when engaged in workshop exercises, but not be so large that the group is swamped. It should be free of exterior distractions and isolated enough so that noise from the workshop does not disturb people outside. Participants are likely to express themselves freely only if it is reasonably intimate and they do not have to keep their voices down.

There must be enough natural light to produce watchable video images, but windows on more than two sides can cause backlighting problems (page 258). Curtains or blinds are helpful to control the light.

An adequate power supply with conveniently placed sockets is needed, and the room must be secure so that equipment can be left in it when the group are working outside.

Finding an appropriate room for the required dates and time can be hard. Less than perfect venues are sometimes unavoidable. However, it is worth persevering as the right space makes creating a supportive workshop atmosphere all the easier.

## Transport

It may be necessary to organize transport so that the participants can get to and from the sessions and so that work can be done on location. Loading and unloading can be a major operation. A driver is useful, particularly if parking nearby is problematic.

## Childcare

It is impossible to take part in a video session and supervise a child at the same time. Childcare must be provided at a sufficient distance from the workshop space so that parents are not distracted.

Parents are frequently unable to attend long sessions and may have little flexibility in their schedules. Workshops should be organized to fit in with school times. Take account of the extra difficulties faced by parents, especially those bringing up children on their own.

## Equipment

Video technology is rapidly evolving and equipment models are constantly upgraded. This can make selecting the appropriate equipment seem a daunting prospect. The main requirements are discussed in Chapter 9.

It normally makes better economic sense to borrow or hire equipment rather than to buy it. In addition, if it is not the right type, or if it breaks down, it can easily be replaced. Certainly do not purchase any equipment until you are completely satisfied that it is suitable.

Vital accessories such as tripods, microphones, headphones and cabling, however, are a worthwhile investment as they can be used with different equipment and are often difficult and relatively expensive to hire.

When choosing video equipment ask for advice, and get several opinions. Information from people who use video in workshop settings is the most relevant.

### Choosing non-standard and adapted equipment

If you are considering using adapted equipment for work with people with disabilities, remember that most modifications are specifically designed. What helps one person can easily hinder another. Before purchasing non-standard equipment, consult the participants themselves.

Wheelchair-mounted camera brackets can sometimes help individual camera operators but they are problematic for group work. They make taking turns on the camera much more time-consuming and they over-emphasize the camera operator's role. A wide angle tripod with no central column, under which a wheelchair can manoeuvre, is often a more satisfactory solution.

Due to the trend towards miniaturization, equipment buttons on camcorders are frequently tiny, posing problems for a range of people, not only those with motor co-ordination difficulties. The positioning of buttons also affects ease of use. Remote controls can assist equipment operation for people with limited hand movement.

## PROJECT MANAGEMENT AND ADMINISTRATION

Every project requires effective management and administration to ensure that it fulfils its aims. The co-ordinator must also support and supervise the workers, keep the funders and other relevant parties up to date with project progress, and control the finances.

## Time

Project management and administration can be time-consuming so make sure that adequate resources are allocated for it. Workers must also allow enough time to plan each session, collect the equipment, set up the workshop, relay feedback and deal with any problems.

## Safety

All group work carries with it responsibility. Make sure that all reasonable safety precautions have been taken and that the work is adequately insured. Workers should be especially careful when working on location (page 127).

## Permission

The participants usually elect to take part in the work themselves. In some cases parents, key workers or centre staff must give permission for participants to join the project because it involves being videoed.

Permission is a more complicated matter when working with certain people, such as prisoners. It may be necessary to get authorization from senior management within the relevant agency.

For example, during a project at a hospital, permission was given to video in the hospital grounds, but the workers had to ensure that no one outside the group appeared on camera, even by accident.

Consent should always be sought before the participants video people outside the group (page 39). If the recorded material is to be shown, or used as part of a programme, it is advisable to obtain written permission.

## Contracts

In certain circumstances written contracts can be drawn up with the project participants. Normally these represent a commitment to attend the sessions, or an agreement to acceptable standards of behaviour, for example agreeing not to drink or smoke in the sessions and to arrive on time.

## Budgeting

The budget for a video project can be divided into two parts: the cost of running the workshop sessions and the cost of organizing the project. The following list covers the main budget items for participatory video work. It does not include any costs relating to producing a final edited tape or organizing a screening.

### Workshop costs

- Video workers' fees
- Video equipment (hire or purchase)
- Video tapes
- Travel expenses for the workers and the group
- Venue hire
- Additional materials and expenses

### Project overheads

- Administration expenses (telephone, photocopying, postage and other sundry office costs)
- Co-ordinators'/management fee
- Staff training
- Insurance for equipment and people
- Equipment maintenance (such as repairing or replacing cables)
- Tape copying
- Report compilation (such as photocopying, photographs and writing-time)

## Evaluation and monitoring

Monitoring provides the means to evaluate the project and improve working practices. If the evaluation is to be effective, monitoring procedures must be agreed before the workshops begin.

In order to monitor the work effectively the aims must be specific. A picture of how the project is proceeding is built up by comparing the activities to the original aims.

It is relatively easy to assess quantitative factors, such as the number of workshops that took place or how many participants attended, but to evaluate the real value of development work, qualitative elements must be appraised. These are more difficult to measure, but information can be gathered in the following ways:

- The workers collect feedback from the participants informally or in a feedback meeting.
- Another member of staff, or an outside evaluator, can visit the project or meet the participants and workers after the sessions.
- The participants can fill out questionnaires or present feedback in a non-written form (e.g. on video).

It is standard practice for a written report to be presented by the workers after the project. Most funders will outline what they require.

# Setting up a project checklist

Consider the following points when setting up a video project.

*Project creation*

- Appropriateness of video.
- Co-ordinator's role.
- Negotiation, consultation, accountability and partnership.
- Taster sessions.

*Project aims*

- Situation and needs.
- Benefits.
- Possible outcomes.
- Suitability of video.
- Achievability of aims.

*Project structure*

Group

- Size.
- Open or closed group.
- Selection procedures.
- Composition.
- Single or mixed experience.
- Appropriateness of issue-based work.

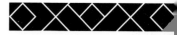

Workers

- Skills, attitude and experience.
- Availability.
- Local knowledge.
- Appropriate for group – shared experience?
- Known to group or not?

Timescale

- Frequency.
- Duration.
- Length of project.

*Project organization*

- Venue.
- Workshop space.
- Transport.
- Childcare.
- Equipment.

*Project management and administration*

- Time for organization and planning.
- Safety.
- Insurance.
- Permission.
- Contracts.
- Finances.
- Evaluation and monitoring.

# Chapter 8

# Developing project plans

This chapter provides a guide to planning project activity. It examines how to structure individual sessions, how to combine different games and exercises to achieve the best results and how to structure a series of workshops.

## DEVELOPMENTAL APPROACH

Participatory video follows a developmental approach. This means that different aspects of the process are developed in parallel throughout the project. Participants do not learn all about video production first, and then afterwards develop the confidence to express their ideas to others. Instead all facets of the work evolve together alongside each other.

The developmental process can be broadly divided into four aspects, as outlined below.

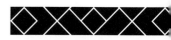

## Individual growth–Group identity–Wider social purpose

Through the project, group members are motivated to participate in activities that cultivate individual development. Taking part encourages mutual support and a sense of purpose. In the group environment they share experiences and find common ground. Co-operation builds a sense of belonging and increases social cohesion. By this process group members can gain confidence to take on new organizational roles and increase their participation in the wider community.

## Expression–Communication–Representation

Video encourages participants to express themselves. They realize that they have things to say, and develop a belief that what they have to convey is of value. As the project progresses they are encouraged to interact with each other and to communicate with other people. Discussing issues and developing ideas stimulates them to represent themselves to others. They organize their opinions, and, as ideas are developed alongside programme-making skills, participants move from expressing something about themselves in simple exercises to devising structured programmes representing their views.

## Skill development–Capacity building–Self-reliance

Participants develop technical, creative and organizational skills by taking part in a series of guided tasks. As the project proceeds they are expected to take more responsibility for all aspects of the work. Through the development of decision-making, planning and evaluation skills, self-determination grows. Group members increase their control over the decisions affecting them and their ability to act.

## Exploration–Questioning–Action for change

Using the equipment as a group to explore their experiences and environment, participants become more aware of their situation. As the process develops they start to evaluate and question the circumstances of their lives and decide what they want to change. By providing a means of voicing their opinions the project can also assist them to bring about controlled changes on a social, organizational, environmental, community or political level.

Not all groups go through every stage of development. The focus depends on the specific needs of the group and the purpose of the project. However, keeping the different aspects of the process in mind can help when making decisions about which exercise to use at any given time.

## WORKSHOP PLANNING

Each workshop forms part of a progressive process. What takes place in a session, its timing and pace, and the amount of worker input varies according to the project goals, the participants' response to the process and the stage in the project.

## Individual sessions

A video workshop follows a fairly standard format. It starts with some introductory or warm-up exercises, which are followed by the main workshop activity. This can be several short exercises, one longer exercise or part of a task spread over several weeks. The session ends with final discussions, conclusions and any plans for the next time the group meets.

While the structure of each workshop is similar, the content varies. Different games and exercises are used to achieve specific results. When choosing games, workers should be clear not only about the aims of the project as a whole but also about the stage of development that the group has reached. At the start of a project, building a sense of community can be important; later on, looking at particular issues in more detail may have greater priority, and is possible because the groundwork has been laid.

Some games are used only once to achieve a particular outcome or to introduce a specific skill; others can be used regularly during a project in different ways. Most sessions start with a simple exercise to refamiliarize the group with video work. Questions in a Row (page 55), for instance, can be used repeatedly to get things going.

Each exercise in a session should relate to the others and lead the group forward. At the same time the exercises should be varied in order to keep the group engaged. Alter the pace throughout the workshop by combining long and short exercises. Use a light-hearted game to break up a period of intense work, or an active game in between periods of inaction. If an exercise takes more than one session to complete, split it at an appropriate point, and recap at the beginning of the next workshop so that everyone understands what is going on.

Each session relates to the general project aims and is part of the ongoing development process, but it is also important to treat it as a discrete entity. It should be self-contained, with no loose ends left hanging for the following session, and it should in itself embody the participatory process. The first and last sessions in particular require special attention.

The workers must both understand the planned activity and be clear about who is to take responsibility for what. You need to reach agreement on respective roles for each exercise to be adequately prepared (page 45). Good communication between co-workers makes it easier to assess the work and solve problems. Evaluate each session, and if it is part of a series of workshops, review the plan in relation to the previous session and adapt it as necessary. Before the project begins it is hard to gauge how fast a group will work, so plan extra exercises as a contingency measure. After a couple of sessions you will have a much better idea of the group's pace.

Your ability to be flexible and responsive to the needs of the group is vital. The plan must be adaptable to allow for variations in the group's reaction. The ability to respond to spontaneity will be helped by careful preparation. Be ready to deal with all eventualities and do not be afraid to change the plan if a good opportunity arises, or if something is not working. A workshop is an interaction between a number of people and as such is a dynamic, organic process.

## Planning a series of sessions

All projects, even short ones, should have a structure. The project plan is developed according to the length and frequency of the sessions, the duration of the project and the nature of the group.

Even in a relatively short project people can benefit considerably from using video. In only five sessions a group can progress from making simple statements expressing opinions to interviewing and constructing programmes.

During a project the challenges increase for the group. As the project unfolds, harder and harder tasks are set and more sophisticated work is undertaken. New roles are introduced and team work is developed.

Structure the project carefully so that a variety of activities takes place and so that it has a distinct beginning and end. The initial sessions are characterized by familiarization. Often this is quite intense and for some participants 30–45 minutes is quite long enough. Groups with short attention spans, such as young children, also require briefer sessions with lots of different exercises to keep them involved.

Many groups start videoing outside from early on; others may require more preparation. Leaving the security of the workshop room to record material on location leads to longer working periods. As the process continues session lengths may need increasing. When the time spent loading, unloading and travelling is taken into account, three to four hours are easily occupied, and some visits can require an entire day.

Activities change and develop during a project to meet the expectations and needs of the group. As a project progresses the options available expand considerably. Drama, documentary, interviewing, storyboarding and location work provide a range of choices. Care must be taken to maintain direction as it is possible to lose sight of the project's purpose amid the enthusiasm.

Video is a talk-based medium so language plays a major part. However, non-verbal versions of many games can be devised for groups who have difficulty talking or hearing.

An initial ten-session project gives an insight into various techniques and programme styles. During the project participants can be provided with a range of experiences so that they are able to make informed decisions about how to continue. For example, they may decide to concentrate on drama and spend time exploring storylines, storyboarding and recording dramatic productions, or they may undertake a more factual approach to production work, planning documentaries and interviewing people outside the group on location.

## EXAMPLE PROJECT STRUCTURE

The following example outlines a structure for a typical ten-session project. The plan is not intended to be definitive but rather provides an insight into the possibilities. It describes how particular games and exercises can be used and highlights some of the issues that can arise when planning a project.

This plan is designed for sessions of about one and a half hours, excluding time for setting up and packing away.

## Workshop 1 – Introductory session

The first session sets the scene for the whole project so it has particular significance. Running an introductory session is explained in Chapter 3.

### Activities

- Name Game
- Questions in a Row
- Chat Show
- Disappearing Game

## Workshop 2 – New skills

The second workshop can be awkward as it frequently lacks the spontaneity and enthusiasm of the first and the structure and concentration of later work. The group is also still getting used to seeing themselves on tape. Keep up the pace but avoid introducing too much information too quickly.

### Activities

- Statements in a Round (e.g. personal news)
- Heads, Hands and Feet
- Commentary Game
- Pop Promo

## Workshop 3 – Moving around

Going out of the workshop space is motivating and can be introduced at this stage with most groups. Use a short exercise to get the group organized before setting off. Then record in the immediate locality, around or just outside the venue, to introduce the activity in a controlled way.

### Activities

- Questions in a Row
- Shot-by-shot Documentary

## Workshop 4 – Presenting information

The group members are encouraged to think about presenting information on video in this session. They then plan what they want to communicate during the news programme. If the group are ready, interviews with other people can be incorporated.

### Activities

- Edited Questions
- Video Whispers
- News Item (with interviews)

## Workshop 5 – Communicating values

This session combines expressive games with exercises involving more planning. Participants develop the confidence to state their opinions. Video Comic Strip introduces them to drama on video.

### Activities

- Statements in a Round (dislikes and likes)
- Personal Advertisement
- Video Comic Strip

## Workshop 6 – Drama and storyboarding

Drama was introduced in the last workshop. Object Mime reintroduces this area of work. The group video a shot-by-shot drama. Use storyboarding if appropriate to add a new dimension to the planning process.

### Activities

- Object Mime
- Shot-by-shot Drama (possibly storyboarded)

## Workshop 7 – Interviews and preparation for going out

Before videoing on location a session is spent consolidating the work undertaken in the project to date. The exercises suggested are used to explore topics, practise questioning and to stimulate co-operation and mutual support. Potential locations to visit in the next session are generated during Statements in a Row.

### Activities

- Opinions
- Grandparent's Footsteps
- In the Hot Seat (in pairs)
- Statements in a Row (about where to video)

## Workshops 8 and 9 – Going out with the group

The best places to visit have several locations within easy reach and some shelter in case of bad weather. When first videoing in public, select a quiet spot to avoid the group being the centre of attention and becoming intimidated. A park or similar public space is excellent.

Going somewhere for refreshments can make the outing more of an occasion. It gives both the participants and the workers a much needed break; it also provides a social dimension and a neutral space to discuss the work.

### Activities

*   Load equipment
*   Shot-by-shot Documentary on location
*   View material back at base

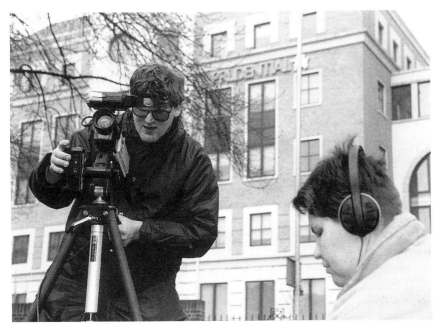

*Figure 8.1* Videoing outside

## Workshop 10 – Conclusion and feedback

Use the final session to review the project, watch the recorded material and discuss what is going to happen after the project is completed. The group need to decide if they want to show any of the material produced. Avoid a sense of anticlimax by continuing the practical work right up to the end.

### Activities

- Questions in a Row (about the project)
- View material, discuss progress made, select material for screening
- Progressive Discussion (about what to do next)
- Discuss future plans

## Ending projects

At the end of a project the group should look forward as well as reviewing what has been achieved. If they want to carry on with video, and this is an option, further plans can be discussed.

There is often work to do after the final session. If the participants want to show their work then a screening can provide a focus for celebration, bringing together other people that have been involved, and generating a real sense of accomplishment and completion. Participants and people outside the group might require copies of the workshop material. These will need to be made and distributed. Workshop tapes should not be reused as the group may want to use their material at a later date. The tapes are their collective work and should be clearly labelled and kept in a safe place.

## Record keeping

The video material itself provides a record of the work done in front of the camera, but the participants themselves must decide which parts of it they want to show; other people must not watch the tape unless participants give consent.

A record of the group using the equipment and working together can be created by taking photographs. These can evoke strong memories of the project and provide a permanent reminder to the group of what they achieved, but taking photographs can be very disruptive and should not happen every session. The participants themselves should decide what type of pictures they want and when they are taken. If an outside photographer visits, make sure that prints will be available for them to keep.

It is useful for workers to keep a project log with comments about what happened during each session. This assists report writing and future planning. It can also be appropriate for the group to write reports or articles about the project. These can be put together with photographs and video material to make an exhibition or to help gain additional project funding.

## PROJECT PROBLEMS AND SOLUTIONS

The difficulties that occur in video projects can be divided into two broad areas: core problems, relating to the participants, the staff and the working practices, and functional problems, associated with the technical, logistical and financial aspects of the work.

## Core problems

Experiential learning is unfamiliar to many people. Taking a more active role than they are used to can make some participants feel insecure. Consequently workers can find themselves pressurized into using a more didactic style because it is what is expected.

Being clear about the project structure helps the group feel more comfortable. Explain at the beginning what they are going to get out of the session, and review what they have achieved at the end.

### Internal hierarchies

Participatory video work is undermined when there is a hierarchy within the group. Hierarchies are frequently supported as much by those who lack confidence as by those who hold the power, because they allow individuals to avoid taking responsibility.

Workers need to deal with the problem as early as possible; power structures are difficult to dislodge once entrenched. It is especially difficult if the group is well established.

Use exercises to develop co-operation and reinforce team work. Make sure that the ground rules are firmly established (page 36), and that opportunities exist for everyone to take part at all levels. Support participation by those people who are being excluded, and do not let individuals dominate the discussion or push others around.

## Dealing with difficult participants

Difficulties with specific individuals in the group can be hard to predict. They can stem from past experiences where competition rather than co-operation was encouraged, or where unhelpful behaviour was the only way that individuals could get attention. Alternatively, individuals can feel that their perceived position within the group is threatened by participatory work. They may try to work against the group process by being overly critical, loudly disinterested or aggressive. An individual who is technically confident may try to assert their authority by undermining other people when they use the equipment.

This type of behaviour is trying and potentially destructive. If it is not resolved quickly it can easily jeopardize the entire project. Involve potential saboteurs by giving them specific responsibilities. If you cannot get them on your side, and peer group pressure has no effect, talk to them about their behaviour and restate the ground rules for taking part. As a last resort individuals may have to be excluded rather than ruin the whole project.

## Conflict of working practice

Other staff who work with the group can cause difficulties when participatory working practices are used, especially when the project is designed to empower the group or bring about organizational changes. Professionals can feel threatened if the project's goals challenge the status quo, particularly if they have not been adequately consulted. Regular discussion and exchange of views is essential. It increases understanding and the staff who are involved are therefore more likely to be supportive.

Nevertheless there may still be genuine disagreement about the approach used in the work or its content. Any differences of opinion should be dealt with well away from the group. Major conflicts or personality clashes can be very hard to resolve, and intervention by someone from outside the immediate situation may be required.

## Functional problems

Any video project can suffer from technical, organizational or financial difficulties at some stage. These problems are often easy to spot but harder to solve.

Small technical problems are annoying; major failure of equipment can lead to delays or cancellation of a project, and is not uncommon. To make technical problems easier to deal with if they arise, identify replacement equipment sources and repair facilities before the project starts.

Even the most carefully organized project can run into logistical difficulties. For instance, rooms get double booked or transport does not arrive. The more that workers are able to predict and minimize potential problems the better.

Raising funding for video projects can be time-consuming and demoralizing; all too often funding for video is made available for capital purchases but not to pay project workers. Under-funding causes stress for the workers and can frustrate participants' development.

Be realistic about the money needed for all aspects of the work, and budget accordingly. Try to raise the entire funding before starting work, and do not agree to do anything that is not covered or cannot be achieved with the available resources. If working to a tight budget, keep an eye on the finances.

## Finding solutions

Problem solving has the following components:

* Recognition
* Analysis and consultation
* Finding, proposing and implementing a solution
* Monitoring effectiveness

The earlier that problems can be identified and addressed, the less risk to the project potential. Often, admitting that something is going wrong is the hardest part.

Finding solutions depends on recognizing the cause. Working out what is happening is not always straightforward. Problem solving is greatly assisted if there is someone outside the situation with whom you can discuss the issues.

Once a solution has been agreed and put into effect the situation should be carefully monitored to make sure that it is resolved. Keep those concerned updated with progress, and take further action as required.

## PLAN FOR SUCCESS

Video projects vary from one-off taster sessions to those lasting several years. Careful planning is essential so that activities support the project purpose.

Plans provide the framework for the developmental process, but they are not rigid structures. They need to be flexible to respond to specific needs, and as the participants determine exactly what happens in a project, outcomes evolve and mature and are rarely quite the same as first envisaged.

Plan for success by being aware of any potential hazards, and create the opportunity for the group to make meaningful choices and have a genuine say in the project's direction.

# Example project plan

### 1 Introductory session

- **Name Game**
- **Questions in a Row**
- **Chat Show**
- **Disappearing Game**

### 2 New skills

- **Statements in a Round**
- **Heads, Hands and Feet**
- **Commentary Game**
- **Pop Promo**

### 3 Moving around

- **Questions in a Row**
- **Shot-by-shot Documentary**

### 4 Presenting information

- **Edited Questions**
- **Video Whispers**
- **News Item (with interviews)**

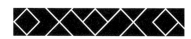

### 5 Communicating values

- **Statements in a Round**
- **Personal Advertisement**
- **Video Comic Strip**

### 6 Drama

- **Object Mime**
- **Shot-by-shot Drama (storyboarded)**

### 7 Interviews and preparation for going out

- **Opinions**
- **Grandparent's Footsteps**
- **In the Hot Seat**
- **Statements in a Row**

### 8 and 9 Videoing on location

- **Shot-by-shot programmes on location**

### 10 Conclusion and feedback

- **Questions in a Row**
- **View material**
- **Discuss progress**
- **Select material for screening**
- **Progressive discussion**
- **Discuss future plans**

# Equipment

# Chapter 9

# Technical teaching and video operation

This chapter covers the technical aspects of participatory video, in order to develop a solid understanding of what video equipment does and how it should be operated.

It considers how to teach technical skills to the participants, suggesting an approach that hands over video production skills in a way that complements the development process. It also explains how to set up and use the equipment for participatory video work.

It is impossible to describe exactly which buttons to press because every video model is slightly different, so basic principles and procedures are presented and details can then be referenced in your equipment manual.

Video production is an enormous subject so this chapter does not attempt to include every aspect. The aim is to cover the operational techniques needed to run the activities described in this book. There is plenty of information available that concentrates solely on production work, should you want to enhance your knowledge and skills.

## TEACHING HANDS-ON VIDEO SKILLS

In participatory video the equipment provides the focus for the group development process. How it is used is central to the success of the work. Through learning how to operate video equipment themselves, participants develop a belief in their own potential, a sense of collective achievement and control over their own agenda.

## Developmental process

Participants do not learn how to use the equipment in isolation. The way that technical skills are transferred is a fundamental part of the development process, inextricably linked to the other aspects. However, teaching the group operational techniques is not the same as the rest of the work. The technical worker develops video production skills on a one-to-one basis, creating an intimate space around the equipment while the other group members prepare. The specific instructions given are not tied to the exercise, or the stage in the project. They depend on individual needs at that moment, as well as the level of the group as a whole. The development of technical skills therefore follows a related but parallel path within the overall process.

This means that video production is not taught to a rigid timetable. Instead, a framework is provided that requires participants to know certain operational procedures. First, basic techniques are introduced, which are then refined on an individual basis. New information is added when appropriate and skills are gradually improved with practice over time.

Parameters are widened in a way that challenges the group to expand their skills without overfacing them. The precise technical knowledge transferred depends on individual requirements, and this allows a quick-learning group to cover more ground than one that finds video operation harder. Nevertheless, the effect of the development process is similar because each group is stimulated by the process of using the equipment in the same way.

## Attitude

Many people are intimidated by video equipment. Often this is a response to social stereotyping (the widely held fallacy that women, older people and other sections of the population are technically inept), or because they were categorized as non-technical at school. If you are told you cannot do something often enough, the message is absorbed, and people can genuinely believe that operating the equipment is beyond them.

The approach to teaching video production is affected by both the participants' and the workers' attitude to technology.

## Participants

The participants' technophobia is manifested in two directions. At one end of the scale, individuals are reluctant to touch the equipment, and extremely over-critical of the results they produce on tape. If their work is not perfect, they take it as proof of their perceived incompetence, even on a first attempt. If there are no mistakes they fabricate them, or refuse to accept that they recorded the tape unaided.

At the other extreme are those who are desperate to appear competent and mask their fear at all costs. Often they fiddle with the equipment at the first opportunity. They press their eye against the viewfinder, and try all the buttons frantically, but cannot take in any information.

Workers must not reinforce a lack of confidence by making assumptions about who is going to be good at using the equipment and who is not. It is very easy to imagine that those who appear to be comfortable touching the equipment already know more than they do. If they miss vital early instruction, it is progressively harder for them to admit to a lack of knowledge.

Feedback also needs careful consideration. In general, participants are all too critical of what they produce. Rather than indicating mistakes, workers should concentrate on counteracting people's tendency to put themselves down. Be encouraging and constructive, pointing out what they have done well to reinforce good work. They will benefit far more from positive criticism.

For example, on a project with a group of older people, one woman watching her camera work declared that she was hopeless because the camera had wobbled and the picture was dark. This was not the time to tell her how to improve. Instead, the worker complimented her on keeping the person in shot when they moved unexpectedly, and explained that the picture went dark because they stepped in front of a window. Later that session an exercise was chosen to clarify backlighting (page 258), so the group learnt through practice without high-lighting an individual's work.

## Workers

The workers' confidence in using the video equipment is vital. If you are unsure about operating it yourself, you are unlikely to inspire the group's faith in their own abilities. Practise until you are comfortable before attempting to teach others.

It is not necessary to be an expert. You can develop your production skills alongside the group, but you must have a sufficient grasp of video technology to facilitate basic equipment operation clearly and keep the equipment safe. Remember that video can break down. Coping with any problems without being thrown, or blaming yourself, is what is needed. If required, spend time familiarizing yourself with video, so that you know what can go wrong, or seek additional training.

It is important that the workers are not too precious about the equipment. The group must be relied on to take care of the equipment themselves. Remember that it was designed to be used. Wear and tear through appropriate use is far better than video equipment sitting in the cupboard awaiting obsolescence. In fact, participants frequently start acting responsibly with the equipment only once they are entrusted with its safety. Confidence with video also helps in handing over responsibility to the participants, as it will make you more aware when intervention is needed to keep things safe, and when you can relax.

## TEACHING APPROACH

People with technical knowledge do not always make good teachers. A thorough understanding of equipment operation is not automatically accompanied by the ability to pass skills on to others. Lack of clarity is frequently compounded by the use of baffling jargon. At worst technicians mystify what they do, making things more complicated than necessary, either because they are unable to explain simply or to exaggerate their status. Remember, anyone can be taught basic video operation with the right support and encouragement. If participants have difficulty, it reflects the instruction they receive more than their ineptitude.

### Learning by doing

Confidence with video equipment increases in direct proportion to hands-on experience. Skills are therefore best learnt through practical activities, not through lectures. The game Heads, Hands and Feet generates comprehension of the space in front of the camera in a way that theory rarely matches (page 76).

Avoid the temptation to demonstrate a procedure. Afterwards each participant still needs individual instruction as they put what they saw into practice. In addition, demonstration increases the emotional barriers that participants must overcome in order to use video themselves, because it asserts your superiority and control over the equipment. If it is really essential that the whole group watches a practical procedure together, teach one person while the others watch.

Workers often make the mistake of showing what they mean by demonstration if their instructions are not understood. The intention is to clarify, but by taking over they give the impression that the participants' attempt was not good enough and feelings of inadequacy are reinforced. Always teach video without touching the equipment yourself. Indicate what to do by pointing or miming. If the person is unsure, you may have to pick up their hand and place it on the equipment, but do not operate it for them.

## Reinforcement through repeated action

Video is mastered experientially through practice by repeating and expanding simple procedures. Do not explain what to do once and expect participants to remember. Instead, aid skill assimilation by following the same process each time you work with an individual. Support the development of their operational abilities by reminding them of the procedure, and by reinforcing it through repetition until the operation becomes second nature. Consistency of language in the way in which technical terms are applied and procedures are ordered will help group members commit them to memory.

## Providing context

Technical operations are introduced most appropriately when they are relevant to the situation. For instance, the first exercise outside provides a good opportunity to explain white balance (page 245). It is given a natural context and participants are more likely to understand it.

The ideal time to bring in a new procedure is when it is initially needed. For instance, the camera operator learns to pan the camera when they have to follow action for the first time (page 246). Prepare tasks that require participants to try out different operations, and provide additional information when it is applicable.

## Participant-led development

Participants should set the pace of technical development. Add new knowledge only when they are ready to take it in.

Participants are likely to be completely engaged in watching themselves on camera early on in the project. The sound may be too quiet, or the picture badly framed, but they will not generally be concentrating on, or even aware of, the technical standard of the recording. They need some experience before they can look at their work more critically. The time to introduce more about microphones is when they ask why they cannot hear properly.

The significance of waiting until participants are ready for new input cannot be over-emphasized. It applies throughout a project, not just at the beginning. It is very easy to overwhelm the group with technicalities beyond their level of perception. Workers, particularly those from production backgrounds, often replay work, picking out everything that needs improving and explaining how to remedy mistakes. The intention is to empower the group by sharing as much technical knowledge with them as soon as possible but unfortunately most of this information goes straight over the participants' heads. They generally are not sufficiently technically aware to comprehend what is being discussed. Frequently eyes glaze over, minds switch off, and they leave reinforced in their belief that video is beyond them.

Of course, new information is not always directly requested by the participants. It is the workers' job continually to widen technical parameters. To help gauge the level of the group's critical awareness you should use questions. This is an important technique. Ask the group what they think of their work and find out what they are pleased with, and what they would like to improve, rather than telling them what is wrong.

## Flexible teaching

Individuals within the group are likely to progress at different rates. The workers must be able to transfer technical skills in a sufficiently flexible manner to respond to each person's level of ability, as well as to the needs of the group as a whole.

Be wary of letting the participants with the most technical knowledge set the pace, or the rest of the group will get lost and their interest will decline. If anyone asks a more complex question do not get drawn into long, complicated explanations. Answer briefly, or tell them that the subject will be covered later, but make sure you set aside time to talk to them individually so they do not feel ignored.

This illustrates the trouble with dealing with technical matters as a group. Teach one-to-one where possible so that participants can learn at their own pace within the wider group context.

## Language

Technical jargon develops because it provides a useful shorthand when professionals communicate with each other, yet it can be misused, reinforcing their expertise whilst alienating outsiders. It does not make technical knowledge accessible.

Avoid overly technical language and jargon, and use plain English to demystify technical procedures. Telling the camera operator to turn a ring to make the picture clear is more explanatory than asking them to focus the camera. Technical terms are best introduced once the participants are more familiar with the equipment, when they can relate them to the practical skills they have acquired.

It is also worth considering body language. Some workers have a tendency to stand next to the equipment and hold on to it as they talk. This can make them feel more confident but it marks their territory, sending the group a strong message about who controls the equipment. Instead, sit down with the group away from the camera, and if you are tall, try not to loom over people when teaching.

## Relationship between co-workers

Co-workers should make sure that they have a consistent approach and divide responsibilities within the session. Think carefully about who teaches the equipment at each exercise. It is a good idea to take turns where feasible so that both workers contribute to all aspects of the work. Nevertheless the gender of the workers may have a bearing. If one is a woman and the other a man it challenges assumptions, and provides a positive role model, if the woman teaches the camera for the majority of the time.

# EQUIPMENT OPERATION

## What is video?

Video is a recording and reproduction system used to store synchronized sound and moving images together on magnetic tape. Particles on the tape are aligned magnetically to represent video and audio signals, and this information is read on playback.

As video technology has evolved, various formats have developed. A video format is defined by the tape size, the quality of the reproduction and the way in which the electronic signals are laid down on tape. Every format records the information differently. Nevertheless, each has features in common.

Audio is normally recorded in linear tracks, as it is on sound tapes; the number of audio tracks varies according to the format. The video signal carries much greater information so a helical scanning system is used. The recording heads spin against the tape direction to increase the relative tape speed, and at an angle to the tape to utilize more of the tape surface. This results in diagonal video tracks (Figure 9.1).

A linear control track is also recorded. This is the electronic equivalent of sprocket holes on film. It provides a pulse to mark the start of each picture frame and to control the speed of playback. In addition some formats record FM (Frequency Modulated) audio multiplexed (combined together) with the video information.

## Basic video equipment

Some understanding of the purpose of each piece of equipment is necessary before using video.

### Camera

The camera's function is to convert the scene into an electronic signal that can be recorded on tape. The light entering the lens is focused on the sensitive surface of a pick-up device (either a charge coupled device – CCD – or a camera tube). A pattern of electrical charges is generated depicting light and dark areas of the picture. This sensor is then scanned or read to produce a fluctuating electrical current representing the image. This is amplified to form the video signal.

### Microphone

In a comparable process the microphone transforms sound into an electronic signal. Sound waves enter the microphone and vibrate a diaphragm. This

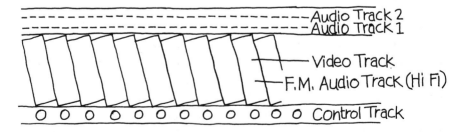

*Figure 9.1* Recording tracks on S-VHS tape

movement generates a minute electrical current that is amplified to become the audio signal.

Video cameras usually have built-in microphones. However, these are not adequate for participatory video work because they pick up sound indiscriminately from every direction. In order to hear what people are saying clearly enough, it is necessary to plug in a separate microphone designed for the specific situation (pages 259–62).

## Video recorder

The video tape recorder (VTR) has two functions. It records the electronic signals produced by the camera and microphone onto the tape, and it reproduces images and sound from pre-recorded tape.

When recording, the video and audio signals are sent to the recording heads, generating an electromagnetic field. As the video tape passes the heads, the magnetic particles are arranged in response to this field. An electromagnetic record of the fluctuating signals is thus created on the tape.

Playback reverses the process. Pre-recorded tape passes the playback heads producing an electromagnetic field. This in turn induces electronic currents which replicate the original video and audio signals.

## Camcorder

A camcorder combines the camera and video recorder in one unit. In this book the term camera includes the camera function of the camcorder and the term recorder the recorder function.

Some camcorders can access camera recording and recorder playback functions at the same time, but often it is necessary to switch between them.

## Monitor

A large colour monitor with a speaker is necessary for participatory video work so that the whole group can see and hear on playback. Although video cameras have black-and-white viewfinders, they are very small, so the separate monitor is also needed for preparation and recording. The camera operator can see clearly, and the bigger image aids facilitation and feedback because it shows the technical worker what the camera operator is doing at all times. The monitor's function is thus to display the video signal during preparation, recording and playback.

The monitor image is produced by an electron beam which scans the monitor's display tube at an intensity determined by the video signal. The phosphor-coated display surface emits light when the electron beam hits it, producing a pattern of light representing the original scene.

Either a video monitor (specifically designed to display a video signal only) or a television can be used, depending on availability and equipment compatibility. A portable battery-powered monitor is useful for outside work.

## Headphones

Headphones monitor the audio signal during preparation and recording. In preference they should have enclosed, plastic-covered ear pieces (not foam only) to cut out as much of the background sound as possible, otherwise the sound recordist can be confused between the microphone sound and the sound coming directly from the surroundings.

## Tripod

The tripod is a three-legged stand to which the camera is attached. It holds the camera securely and is vital for steady, professional-looking video work. It also makes teaching and learning easier and creates a base around which the group can work.

## Power adapter and charged batteries

Video equipment is powered by mains electricity but it is not plugged in directly. A power adapter transforms the mains AC supply to the much smaller DC voltage needed by the equipment. When working off the mains, extension leads and multiple socket adapters may also be required.

Batteries power the equipment when the mains supply is not accessible. One battery supplies the recorder and the camera. Video batteries are reusable and they must be charged up ready for the session. The power adapter generally functions as a charger when it is not running the equipment.

## Cabling

Cabling is needed to attach the equipment together. Check that all the required leads are supplied.

## *Blank video tape*

Video tape is made from a flexible polyester material coated with easily magnetized metal oxide. It is housed in a cassette. The kind of video tape cassette required depends on the format and type of equipment. The most common domestic formats are VHS, S-VHS, Video 8 and Hi-8. The S-VHS and Hi-8 formats are higher-quality versions of VHS and Video 8. VHS or Video 8 tape can be used in S-VHS and Hi-8 equipment respectively but the better quality is sacrificed. Some VHS and S-VHS equipment uses compact tapes (VHS-C and S-VHS-C), so check whether you need the full or compact size.

To protect tapes from being accidentally erased, most cassettes have a record tab to remove, or a switch to slide, which prevents recording (page 252).

## SELECTING EQUIPMENT TO USE

To run a participatory video project the following equipment is required:

- Camera and video recorder or camcorder
- Separate microphones
- Large monitor and portable battery-powered monitor
- Headphones
- Tripod
- Power adapter and charged batteries
- Extension leads and cabling
- Blank video tape
- Carrying cases for equipment

This list defines the basic minimum. It is possible to manage without a portable monitor but outside work is improved considerably if one is available.

## Format

You are most likely to have access to VHS, S-VHS, Video 8 or Hi-8. VHS has the advantage that it can be played back on most home VTRs. Opting for a higher-quality format depends on money, but if the plan is to produce work to distribute widely it is advisable. Newer digital tape formats, such as DVC, will also be worth considering as they become more available, particularly as editing machines are developed.

## Separate equipment

A separate camera and recorder are preferable to a camcorder for group work. If the two functions are combined in one unit too much control is invested in the operator and it is harder for more than one person to access the equipment at a time. Camcorders are far more common but it is better to use separated equipment if possible.

## Size

The lightest video equipment is not necessarily the most suitable. Camcorders often have tiny buttons that are difficult to see and fiddly to operate. Very small equipment is also more fragile. Consider these factors alongside portability.

## Functions

Video equipment can be covered with buttons offering extra features of little practical use. When choosing equipment it is more important to ensure that basic functions are included and easily accessible.

### Camera

Avoid equipment without manual zoom and focus. Manual white balance and iris control are a bonus.

### Recorder

The equipment must have a separate microphone input and a headphone socket to be suitable for participatory video. Try to find a recorder that can audio-dub and has manual audio-level controls.

### Microphones

A separate hand-mike is sufficient initially. A directional mike has many uses. Lapel mikes and boundary mikes are more specialized (page 259). For workshops, very expensive microphones are not normally required; it is more important to use the right type.

## *Tripod*

Use a tripod designed for the weight of the camera/camcorder. Braces hold the legs together and increase security when the tripod is in use, and rubber feet stop slippage. A fluid head, which assists smooth panning and tilting of the camera, is great but not essential.

## WIRING UP

The thought of wiring up the equipment deters many people from using video. Being faced with several bits of equipment and a pile of leads can be quite daunting if it is not familiar. Do not worry – this is a common reaction and it really is not as complicated as it looks.

The specifics of wiring up vary with every video model. Remember the function of each piece of equipment and follow the step-by-step process below (Figure 9.2). This will enable you to tackle various pieces of video equipment and isolate the source of any problems yourself.

Allow plenty of time if wiring up is unfamiliar. If you start to panic, take a deep breath, and think logically through each step. Remember that video equipment is not designed to blow up if a lead is attached incorrectly. Compare the ends of the leads with the sockets on the equipment. As long as a connector is not forced into a hole it does not fit, it is unlikely to do any damage.

## For use on mains power

Position the equipment for the session (page 42). Put the monitor, power adaptor and separate recorder on a table, and set the tripod up next to it. If the ground is flat make sure that the tripod legs are the same length before spreading them out. Some tripods have a spirit level for use when the ground is uneven. Adjust the tripod plate so that it is horizontal and then lock all movement so that the tripod is stable.

Connect the camera/camcorder. Frequently it screws directly onto the tripod plate. Sometimes the plate itself is detachable and screws onto the base of the camera. The camera and plate then clip together onto the tripod. Always double check that the camera is securely attached before letting go of it.

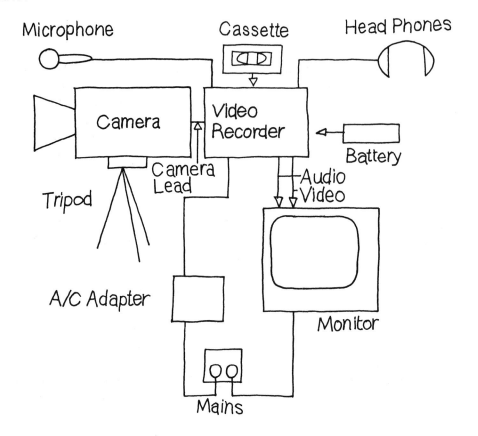

*Figure 9.2* Wiring diagram

### Video and audio

Next the video and audio signals need to be routed round the system. The video signal from the camera is first sent to the recording heads. A camcorder does this internally. With separate equipment, attach the camera to the recorder with the camera lead. This lead is easily recognizable because its connectors have lots of pins or holes. Compare the connectors to the equipment to discover where they go.

Sound enters the equipment via the microphone. Plug it into the external microphone socket, which is usually found on the recorder and labelled. The separate mike generally over-rides the built-in camera mike, but check this is so. Then plug the headphones into the socket on the recorder labelled 'headphones', 'phones', or marked with an ear symbol.

Finally the video and audio signals are routed from the recorder to the monitor. The leads used depend on whether you use a video monitor or an ordinary television.

## Video monitor

A video monitor generally requires two leads, one for the audio and one for the video. Think about the direction in which the signal is travelling. Connect the video lead from 'Video Out' on the recorder to 'Video In' on the monitor, and the audio lead from 'Audio Out' on the recorder to 'Audio In' on the monitor. Sometimes the monitor uses only one lead to carry both the audio and the video.

## Television

Televisions are designed to receive RF (radio frequency) signals not video signals. However, most domestic video equipment contains an RF unit which combines the video and audio, converting them into a higher frequency RF signal that can be picked up by a television.

To connect the recorder to a television use an RF lead (like the one used between a home VTR and the television). Plug it from 'RF Out' on the recorder or the power unit to 'RF In' at the back of the television (the aerial socket).

Camcorders sometimes have a separate RF unit. Attach a lead from the camcorder to the unit, and from the unit to the television.

You will probably need to tune the television to the video recorder after the equipment is powered up, particularly if it is the first time they are used together (see switching on, below).

## Television/video monitor

Some televisions also function as video monitors on the audio/video channel. Wire up as for a video monitor and turn to the relevant channel.

## Power

Each piece of equipment must be connected to a power supply. Fully unwind the extension lead (page 245), and plug it into the wall socket. Plug in the power adapter (checking that it is switched to operate rather than to charge). Then connect the power adapter to the recorder. (If using separate equipment, power travels from the recorder to the camera along the camera lead.)

The monitor is plugged directly into the mains. Finally the microphones; some work without power (particularly hand-mikes) but others need a battery. Take microphones batteries out for storage but do not forget them when you collect the equipment.

## Working on batteries

When powering the equipment using batteries rather than mains power, the power adapter and the extension lead are not required. Instead simply plug a charged battery into the recorder. A separate battery is also needed for the portable monitor.

The battery-powered monitor is connected to the recorder in the same way as a large monitor, and wiring up is the same as on mains in every other respect.

## Charging batteries

Video batteries do not last long. Twenty minutes recording is a usual maximum. Conserve power where possible, and make sure that you charge enough batteries for the session.

The power adapter is generally used to charge batteries. Check the instruction manual for details. Nickel-cadmium (NiCad) batteries should be stored discharged, and recharged before use. They should always be discharged fully before recharging, or they may lose their full capacity. Lead-acid batteries should be recharged after use, and stored charged.

# PREPARATION

## Switching on

Switch on the mains supply followed by each piece of equipment. Do not forget the microphone. Some equipment has more than one operating switch so check that everything is on, and disengage standby mode.

Take the lens cap off. The camera image is displayed on the monitor, as long as the iris is open (page 258). If there is a picture in the camera viewfinder only, the monitor may need switching to the correct input or tuning in. With a television try changing channels first. If there is no success, pick a channel, play a pre-recorded tape in the recorder, and tune the television to the recorder signal in the same way as it is tuned to a television signal. Video monitors do not need tuning so just switch to select the input. Remember to keep the monitor sound turned down except when playing back to avoid feedback.

Listen to the headphones to check sound, and then do a test recording (page 253). If there is a problem, think logically through the wiring process, and recheck relevant leads. Wiggling their ends can reveal a bad connection. (It is worth carrying a spare set of leads as connections do loosen with use.)

Finally, white balance the camera to complete preparation.

## White balance

Different light sources produce differently coloured light. For instance, indoor light from light bulbs has a yellow tinge, while outdoor light from the sun is bluer. The human eye adapts automatically to these differences, but the camera must be adjusted electronically for the prevailing light conditions to reproduce colours correctly.

A filter system for indoor, outdoor and fluorescent light is often provided for rough adjustments. Better results are produced by white balancing.

To white balance manually, point the camera at a white surface with light falling on it, or use a white lens cap. Press the 'white balance' button until the camera indicates that the process has finished. Watch the monitor to see the colours change. The reds, blues and greens in the picture are balanced out so that white looks white.

White balancing should be performed at each new location and whenever the light conditions change (e.g. if the sun goes behind a cloud or is rising or setting).

Most camcorders white balance automatically but manual adjustments produce better colours in more difficult conditions. Avoid mixed light sources, such as indoor light combined with outdoor light from the window, which is hard for the equipment to cope with.

## SAFETY AND EQUIPMENT CARE

To protect the video equipment and work with it safely:

- Make sure that all mains leads are wired up correctly, and that all plugs have the correct size of fuse.
- Always fully unwind extension leads. If they are used only partially unwound, they can overheat.
- Never overload the mains supply. In the UK one socket can power a maximum of about 3,000 Watts, and the ring main about 7,000 Watts (less if you use a long extension lead). This becomes a real issue when using lights when three 800 Watt lights and the rest of the video equipment is generally too much for one socket.
- Protect the equipment from physical bangs, dust and wet. Avoid subjecting it to extreme heat, cold or humidity, or to an abrupt change from cold to heat which produces condensation. Switch off and disconnect during an electrical storm.
- Do not cover the equipment or block its ventilation or it will overheat.
- Keep the lens cap on the camera between shots and when moving around.

Do not touch the lens. Clean it with a lens brush, or lens cleaning paper and fluid. Never wipe a dry lens.

- The lens acts as a magnifying glass, focusing the entering light onto the pick-up device. Older tube cameras can be damaged beyond repair by pointing them at the sun or strong lights, so never do this. CCDs are unlikely to be damaged by normal operating conditions but avoid prolonged exposure to bright light sources such as the sun.
- To move around safely, gather up all the leads so nothing is trailing, and make sure that people carrying attached equipment walk together. Cross roads carefully as a group.
- Avoid jerking the cables.
- Invest in carrying cases to protect the equipment.

## USING THE EQUIPMENT

### Setting up the camera

The camera defines the image that is recorded on tape. A picture is displayed in the viewfinder and on the monitor as soon as the equipment is switched on, not just when recording. The camera operator uses it to assist shot preparation before recording begins.

The image can be altered by physically moving the camera in relationship to the subject. The closer the camera the more the subject fills the frame, and conversely more fits in the frame from further away.

Continuously moving the camera position is inconvenient so the image can be modified in other ways.

### The tripod

The tripod legs are extended or shortened to adjust the camera height. In addition it is often possible to gain extra height by racking up a central column. Alter the legs in preference to avoid the tripod becoming top-heavy, and always make sure they are fully spread.

The camera is attached to the tripod's panning head. This allows it to be swivelled and tilted. Tilting points the camera down towards the floor or up towards the ceiling. Panning moves it in a sideways, horizontal arc. Locks are used to secure and release these movements.

## The camera lens

Video cameras are fitted with zoom lenses as standard. A zoom lens can be adjusted from wide angle to telephoto. Zooming in to the telephoto end of the lens range brings the subject closer, increases its size, compresses depth and reduces the amount of background in the frame. Zooming out makes the subject appear smaller and further away, exaggerates perspective and reveals more of the background.

The zoom lens is adjusted manually using a zoom arm on the lens barrel, or by using a rocker switch to control a powered motor drive. Motorized zooming drains power so zoom manually to set up shots, particularly on battery.

## Focusing

Most video cameras have an automatic focusing system. Turn it off for participatory video work. This is for two reasons. Firstly, automatic focus has limitations. Certain systems cannot cope with smooth shiny surfaces, low contrast or dark subjects. They can be confused about what to focus on, targeting the centre of the screen when the subject is actually off-centre, or a foreground such as a fence or glass, and sometimes go irritatingly in and out of focus as they search for a target.

Secondly, learning to focus the camera manually increases the participants' contact with the equipment and their control over the images produced. Manual focusing involves preparing focus for each shot before recording starts. It follows a simple routine that soon becomes second nature:

- Select subject.
- Loosen tripod.
- Zoom in.
- Focus.
- Zoom out and frame shot (Figure 9.3).

If the subject selected is a seated person, first loosen the tripod so that the camera can pan and tilt freely. (Remember to hold the tripod arm when the tripod is unlocked.)

Next zoom in on the subject's face. You do not need to see the whole face to focus. Go in as close as possible, to the extreme telephoto end of the lens, concentrating on the eyes.

Turn the focus ring at the front of the lens until the image is sharp. Use the large monitor, rather than the viewfinder, for feedback because it is bigger and clearer.

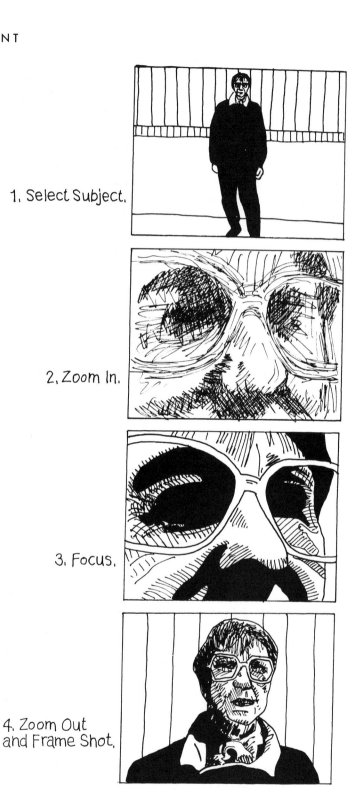

1. Select Subject.

2. Zoom In.

3. Focus.

4. Zoom Out
and Frame Shot.

*Figure 9.3* Focusing

Finally, zoom out and frame the shot. Do not touch the focus ring again. As long as the distance between the subject and the camera stays constant, the image remains in focus zoomed in or out for the following reason.

When a particular position in front of the lens is in focus, a certain distance behind and in front of it is also reasonably sharp. This distance from front to back is known as the depth of field. When zoomed in, the depth of field is at its smallest, so focusing is most critical. This is why the camera is best focused at the telephoto end of the lens. If the picture is in focus zoomed in, it remains so as the camera zooms out because the depth of field increases. However, if the camera is focused at the wide angle end of the lens and then zoomed in, the subject is likely to go out of focus as the depth of field decreases.

## Framing

After focusing, frame the image by tilting, panning and zooming. Remember that if the camera and subject are repositioned you must refocus. When the shot is framed, tighten the tripod for stability, except when the camera needs to follow action.

## Setting up the sound

There are two ways to monitor the audio signal. The headphones are used to assess sound quality and the audio-level meters to evaluate sound levels.

Listen to the headphones to check that the microphone is picking up the sound required and nothing else. Assess whether it is clearly audible, and ensure that the background sound is not too loud or distracting. If there is a problem, check that the mike is close enough to the sound source, is pointing the right way and is the right type for the situation.

Sound leads can get unplugged and microphones switched off. Make sure that the sound can be heard in the headphones. Sound leads also suffer from being pulled around and can develop loose connections, resulting in buzzes, hums or intermittent sound. If the sound fails, even when recording, the sound recordist should stop the action.

The sound level is monitored using the audio meter and adjusted with the level control (Figure 9.4). A moving needle indicates the peaks in sound level. Its position is adjusted so that it is as high as possible without the needle going constantly into the red region on the meter (Figure 9.5). When the needle is in the red, the sound will be distorted.

The sound level goes up and down continuously. Aim to set an average level for the situation. Do not alter the levels all the time or the background sound will

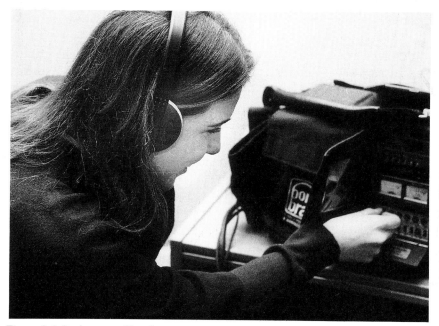

*Figure 9.4* Setting sound levels

keep changing. Do not worry if the needle occasionally peaks in the red. This is better than the overall level being too quiet.

Most camcorders do not have audio meters or manual level controls. The headphones must be used to assess the sound level and to listen for distortions, and the only way to alter the levels is to move the mike.

## Operating the recorder

### *Loading and unloading video tape*

Most equipment needs power to load and unload video tape, so first switch on. Then press 'eject' to open the recorder.

Check that the tape in the cassette is wound tightly, particularly if using compact-sized tapes. (Some cassettes have a gear on the casing that takes up tape slack when turned.)

Insert the cassette with the label side outermost and the arrow pointing into the machine. Then close the recorder gently.

To unload first press 'stop'. This unlaces the tape from around the recorder heads (see below). Press 'eject' and slide out the cassette.

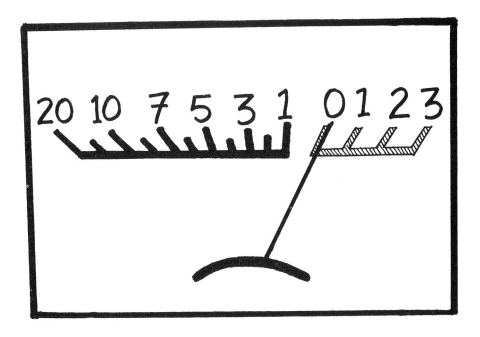

Indicates Red On Dial

*Figure 9.5* Typical audio meter

## Playback functions

Press 'play' to watch the tape. The tape is first taken out of the cassette and wound around the playback heads. As it plays forward anything pre-recorded on the tape is displayed in the viewfinder and on the monitor. A blank tape looks like snow (black with white dots and dashes). Listen to the sound on the headphones, or turn up the monitor sound.

If the pictures are 'snowy' or 'noisy', try adjusting the tracking control. If the pictures are blurred or disappear sporadically, the tape heads may need cleaning (refer to the instruction manual or a video service centre).

Press 'stop' on the recorder to finish watching. Use 'fast-forward' (FF) or 'rewind' (REW) to wind the tape at speed forwards or backwards respectively (Figure 9.6).

Pressing 'pause' after 'play' stops the tape playing forwards, but keeps the tape laced around the playback heads, so that a still picture is shown on the monitor. In a similar way, using 'fast-forward' or 'rewind' after 'play' maintains the tape lacing, so that pictures are displayed as the tape is searched forwards or

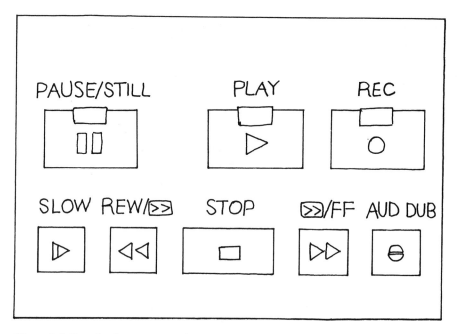

*Figure 9.6* Function buttons on typical recorder

back. Using this search mode is the easiest way to locate the start or end of an exercise.

### Preparing to record

First play the tape to see what it contains, so that nothing important is accidentally erased. Wind on past any pre-recorded material, and pause the tape at the point at which you want recording to start. Then set record mode. Record mode positions the tape against the recording heads so it is ready to record but paused.

Setting record mode varies according to the equipment. Sometimes 'pause' and 'record' are pressed together; or 'pause', 'record' and 'play'; or 'record' only. Camcorders often set record mode when they are switched from the playback to the record function. Check the instruction manual for details.

Always set record mode after pausing in the right place on the tape. Do not press 'stop'. If 'stop' is pressed instead of 'pause', the tape is disengaged from the recording heads (page 250) and rewound back into the cassette. If record mode is then set, the tape is further back than the selected position, and pre-recorded material can easily be erased when recording starts.

If the equipment will not enter record mode, check that the cassette's record tab has not been removed or switched to prevent erasure (page 239). If so, stick a piece of tape over the space, or reposition the tab.

## Recording

Once the equipment is in record mode simply press the main record button on the camera to start recording. It is usually large and red and located near the camera hand-grip. An indicator in the viewfinder, and a red light on the camera, are generally displayed when recording. Press the record button again to stop recording.

## Replaying

To replay, first press 'stop' to disengage record mode. Then press 'play' and use 'rewind' to search for the start of the recording. 'Pause' while the monitor is positioned and the sound turned up. Then disengage 'pause' to watch the tape.

## Test recording

To check that everything is working a test recording can be performed. Set up the camera and microphone. Prepare to record, record 20–30 seconds with sound, and then stop and replay.

## Stepping down

If the equipment is left in record mode for longer than a predesignated time (usually about five minutes), then it will step down. The recorder takes itself out of record mode to prevent wear to the tape and the heads. If the equipment has stepped down, nothing happens when the record button is pressed. Always check it is in record mode before counting in.

## PRODUCTION

### Recording shots

The camera, sound and action are prepared before recording. The floor manager counts in only once everything is ready (page 57). Next, recording is started.

After the required time the camera is switched off again. The result recorded on tape constitutes the shot.

## Recording time lag

If action or speech begins immediately the record button is operated, the first second or two is not recorded. A time lag exists between pressing the record button and the start of recording while the equipment responds to the instruction. Performers must allow for recording time lag by waiting a few seconds before beginning. The floor manager can cue them in.

Recording time lag varies from machine to machine. To work it out for your equipment, point the camera at a clock face with a second hand. Set up record mode, and press record when the second hand is at an exact position, such as when it hits twelve. Stop and replay. The difference between the second hand's position on the first recorded frame and when record was pressed is the time lag for the equipment.

# In-camera editing

In-camera editing involves building up shot sequences directly onto the tape.

## Recording one shot after another

After recording one shot on the tape, the equipment remains in record mode, as long as the stop button is not pressed. Another shot can be recorded directly after the first, by repositioning the camera and then starting recording again. The second shot follows on from the first without any breaks or picture disturbance.

## Setting the recorder up in record mode at a specific place on the tape

The recorder is often stopped between shots, for instance to save power when moving to a new location, to rewind and play the tape, or because the recorder has stepped down (page 253). If it has been stopped it needs to be set up in record mode again at a precise position on the tape, so that the next shot is linked to the preceding one.

Play the tape and pause it at exactly the point where the new shot should start. Then set record mode (see backspace edit below), so that it is ready to start recording from this point onwards. Remember to use 'pause' rather than 'stop' when selecting position to ensure that the tape does not rewind into the cassette (page 252).

The same technique is used to set up to re-record over an unsatisfactory shot.

## Backspace edit

Most recent equipment has a backspace edit function to ensure clean editing between one shot and the next. To avoid the tape rolling back when record mode is set, and erasing part of the previous shot when recording starts, hold down 'pause' throughout record mode set-up (check manual for details).

## Standby mode

Keeping the equipment in record mode between shots drains the batteries. In any case, if the next location is some distance, or the shot takes a while to prepare, the recorder is likely to step down (page 253). However, setting up record mode to link shots after the tape has stopped is time-consuming and fiddly.

Some equipment has a standby mode which conserves power by supplying only essential functions. When power is returned the recorder is still in place for the next shot, which greatly assists in-camera editing.

## Recording black on tape

A blank tape plays back as snow (page 251). When creating shot sequences it looks messy cutting from snow to the first shot of a sequence, or from the last shot back to snow. The solution is to record a totally black picture before the first and after the last shot.

Set up record mode. Put a black lens cap on the camera, and unplug or turn off the microphone. Record 10 seconds or more. As the lens cap prevents any light entering the lens the picture appears completely black.

Remove the lens cap and record the shot sequence. Then, after the last shot, put the lens cap on and repeat.

## Assemble and insert editing

Editing takes place electronically in two ways. The technique used predominantly when in-camera editing is called assemble editing. One shot is recorded after the next on the tape, as described, replacing any previously recorded video, audio and control track.

Assemble editing has disadvantages. Pictures and sound are always recorded together, and the sequence must be recorded in order from first to last shot. It is not possible to go back and replace a shot in the middle of a sequence, because any previously recorded material on the tape is erased when assemble editing, before the new signals are recorded; and as the erase head is physically in advance of the record head, a gap is created on the tape after the assemble edit. If the edit is in the middle of a shot sequence, some of the following shot is erased and the sequence is ruined by the blank gap (Figure 9.7).

Insert editing allows new pictures and sound to be inserted over pre-recorded material to replace the signals. It is usually possible only in an edit suite. The control track from the original material is maintained and used to control the edit very precisely. Editing does not have to be sequential because the original control track is not replaced and so no blank gap is created on the tape. It is also possible to insert video or audio only (Figure 9.7).

Insert editing works over pre-recorded material only. Before editing in an edit suite the master tape is blacked, by recording a black signal from the start to the end of the tape, to supply a continuous control track for editing control.

## Audio-dub

Audio-dubbing is a form of insert editing (Figure 9.7) that some production equipment can do. In audio-dub one or both of the linear audio tracks are replaced with a new sound-track. It is used for adding commentary, music or sound effects.

To prepare to audio-dub, search the tape and pause it before the visuals that

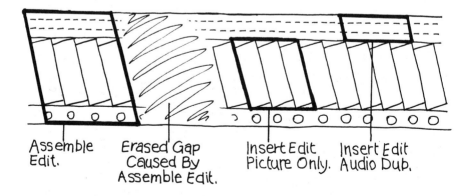

Assemble Edit.    Erased Gap Caused By Assemble Edit.    Insert Edit Picture Only.    Insert Edit Audio Dub.

*Figure 9.7* Assemble and insert editing

need new sound. Then set audio-dub mode (see equipment manual). This is frequently the same as setting record mode except that 'audio-dub' is pressed instead of 'record'. The recorder is then ready to audio-dub from this point onwards.

To start, play the tape, and sound from the microphone replaces the original audio signal (Figure 9.8). During audio-dub the visuals are displayed on the monitor so that commentary can be matched to the pictures. At the end of the sequence pause the tape, and then press 'stop' to disengage audio-dub mode.

Like all insert editing, audio-dub works only over pre-recorded material with a control track. If there are any gaps in the visuals, audio-dub mode will disengage.

If your equipment is able to audio-dub, check which audio track is replaced, and plug the microphone into the correct socket. Make sure that any sound you want to keep is originally recorded on the other track or as FM audio.

## Picture insert editing

Some production equipment provides a picture insert facility, which enables a new video signal to be inserted over previously recorded material whilst

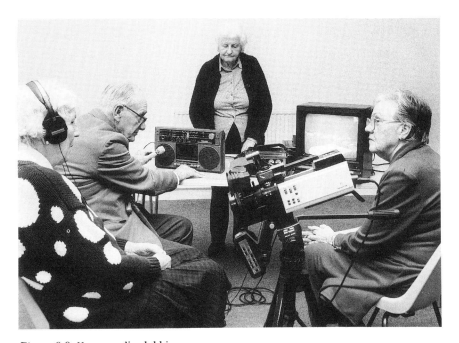

*Figure 9.8* Group audio-dubbing

maintaining the original sound-track. In practice this function is difficult to use accurately when in-camera editing.

## LIGHTING

A video image is correctly exposed when the most important tones are clearly reproduced. If there is too little light, the image is dark and noisy. If there is too much light, the colours are pale and washed out.

### The iris

Exposure is controlled by the iris. Video cameras have automatic irises. If the scene is bright, the iris closes down to let less light in, and if dark, it opens up.

An automatic iris is convenient in most situations. Nevertheless they are designed for an average environment and sometimes create problems. For instance, the exposure fluctuates when the camera pans from light to shade, or as a large object passes by in front of the lens, such a bus driving past close to the camera.

If your equipment has manual iris control, use it to make minor adjustments when necessary.

### Backlight

An area of strong light directly behind the subject, such as a window, or expanse of bright sky, is called backlight. The automatic iris adjusts to the average level of light in the whole picture. The backlight is much brighter than the subject, so the iris shuts down, making the subject very dark.

Some cameras have a backlight switch. This opens up the iris in an attempt to remedy the situation. A manual iris can produce the same effect. However, these adjustments compensate only to a certain extent because video cannot deal with the large contrast ratio between the backlight and the subject.

Instead, avoid backlit images wherever possible. Move the camera, or the subject. If this is not feasible, zoom in to a close-up to reduce the backlight to a minimum.

## Light levels

Video requires plenty of light to produce sharp pictures and good colour. Nonetheless, extra lights are best avoided for several reasons:

- They make the recording environment more intimidating. This increases the pressure on participants when the aim is to relax them.
- They are time-consuming to set up, slowing down the production process considerably.
- They create a more hazardous working environment.

Make the most of the available light and change position in preference to using additional lighting. Also remember the purpose of the work. It does not matter if workshop material is darker than ideal, as long as the pictures are visible. Extra lights are essential only when producing final products for distribution.

## Video lighting

If additional lights are needed, three 800 Watt video lights are a suitable minimum (Figure 9.9). The key light (main light source) is placed to the side of the camera from high up. A fill light is then positioned at about 45 degrees to the first to fill in shadows. The fill light should be less intense, so reflect the light from a flat surface, such as the ceiling, or a specially designed reflector; alternatively, use a diffusing filter in front of the light. Then set up a backlight, pointing towards the back of the subject's hair (not into the camera lens), to bring them away from the background. If you have a fourth light it can be used to light the background itself.

Light from a window can function as the key or fill light, but use daylight-blue filters over the other lights so that all the light sources are a consistent colour and the lighting is not mixed (page 245).

## SOUND

## Microphones

The type of microphone used determines the area from which sound is picked up. Microphones are defined by their pick-up pattern (Figure 9.10).

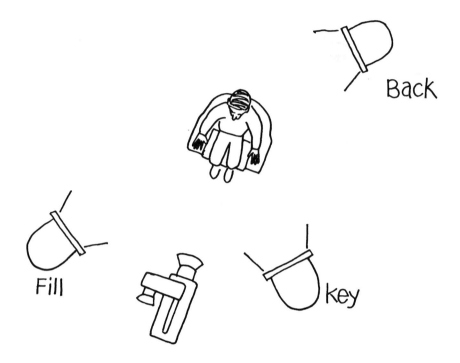

*Figure 9.9* Lighting diagram

## Hand-mike

A hand-mike picks up sound to a distance of about 0.6m (2ft), after which it cuts off quite sharply. It records voices clearly, even when there is background noise. It appears in shot so it is not suitable for drama.

For best results hold the hand-mike 15–46cm (6–18in) from the mouth. It is slightly directional so aim it towards the person speaking. Alternatively, hold it still between two people sitting close, to cut down handling noise (see below).

## Directional mike

A directional (shot-gun) microphone picks up sound predominantly in one direction. The degree of directionality depends on the particular mike. It is used out of shot for documentaries, drama and background sound.

Aim it at the sound you want to record. It must be pointed accurately at the sound source for best results.

When working in front of a busy road the mike can pick up the person

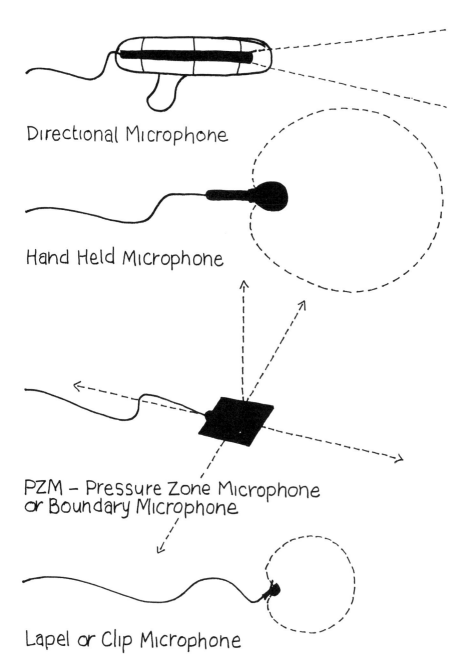

Directional Microphone

Hand Held Microphone

PZM – Pressure Zone Microphone
or Boundary Microphone

Lapel or Clip Microphone

*Figure 9.10* Microphone pick-up patterns

speaking and the cars behind them. To avoid this, direct it from low down, towards the person's mouth and the sky beyond.

Directional mikes are often mounted on a boom arm, and held over the action, particularly for drama. Adapt a broom handle as a cheap alternative.

### Lapel mike

A lapel (personal/tie-clip) mike has a similar pick-up pattern to a hand-mike. It is used by presenters for statements to camera.

Fasten it to clothing, about 15–23cm (6–9in) from the mouth, hiding the lead as much as possible.

### Boundary mike

A boundary (PZM) mike balances sound from different distances so that it is about the same level. It is used for discussions, conference presentations and drama.

The mike is attached to a square plate. Put it on a flat surface, such as a table, or attach it to a smooth wall or a scenery flat. The surface needs to extend at least 1m (3ft) around the mike for best results.

## Noise problems

### Handling noise

Handling noise is picked up when the microphone and cable are touched or moved. Some microphones are more prone to handling noise than others. Hold microphones as still as possible when recording, and try not to disturb the cable.

### Wind noise

Wind produces a low-frequency roaring sound even on a relatively still day. All microphones need wind protection for outside work. The simplest are foam covers that slip over the mike. More expensive wind-shields suspend the mike against vibration in a basket, covered in a furry muffle.

## Sound channels

Most low-budget video equipment has one external microphone socket that inputs the same sound onto all the audio tracks. Better-quality equipment has more than one socket, so that all available tracks can be utilized.

If both linear tracks are available, use audio-track one for main sound and audio-track two for background sound on VHS and S-VHS. Audio-track one is on the inside of the tape and less prone to tape damage. (The positions are reversed with some formats.)

If the equipment offers FM audio, the sound is generally recorded on the FM tracks and the linear tracks at the same time. If not, consider carefully which to use, as the FM sound is interlinked with the video, which can cause problems when audio-dubbing or editing.

# IMAGE COMPOSITION

## Rule of thirds

Traditionally, visual images are thought to look better if they divide the picture into thirds vertically and horizontally. The subject, the eye-line, or any obvious features should be placed a third of the way across, or up, the screen rather than centrally.

Sky is an exception on video. If the skyline is a third of the way down the screen, the image is likely to be backlit, so reduce sky to a minimum.

## Framing

Framing should not restrict the subject. Leave enough room around the subject's head, avoiding chins on the bottom of the screen and foreheads bashing the top. Also, leave looking space if the subject is facing sideways, and space to move into if they are in motion.

However, the subject will look lost if there is too much room around them. Frame reasonably tightly to concentrate the viewer's attention.

## Distracting objects

Avoid plants, telegraph poles or other distracting objects that appear to grow out of the subject's head or shoulders.

## Shot sizes

Shot sizes are defined according to the proportion of the subject contained in the frame. Long-shots, mid-shots and close-ups are the basic shot categories (Figures 9.11a and 9.11b). They are not exact divisions but aid communication during production planning.

## Camera angles

The camera height changes the camera angle. Positioning the camera at eye-level to the subject is neutral. If the camera looks down at it, it looks weak and vulnerable. If it looks up at the subject, it looks imposing, threatening or powerful. Setting up the tripod for operating convenience only may create these effects inadvertently.

## Perspective

A lens with a standard focal length produces the same perspective as the human eye. The zoom lens on a video camera is normally standard at the wide-angle end of the zoom. Therefore shots look more natural if the camera is closer to the subject, rather than zoomed in from a distance. In addition, working at the wide-angle end of the lens makes focusing less critical, and the effect of any camera shake is reduced.

Telephoto flattens perspective, squashing the subject against the background, and making movement appear slow. Use it to create crowd scenes. A true wide-angle lens (wider than the wide-angle end of the zoom) exaggerates perspective, emphasizes depth and space and is more dramatic. Use it to fit more background into the frame, or to emphasize foreground gestures, but remember it can distort the subject.

## Camera movement

Keep the camera still most of the time, letting the action in the scene provide the movement. Wandering camera work, that looks jerkily around and zooms randomly in and out, is not easy to watch or to edit. Conventionally the aim is that viewers see the image created, not the camera's presence.

The main function of the zoom lens is in shot preparation. If you must zoom when recording, do so extremely sparingly and with good reason. Also refrain from panning across a still scene.

Panning to follow action works because it reproduces the way in which the eye locks onto movement and follows it. The picture movement also helps to disguise any camera vibration.

Tracking involves the camera moving position in relation to the scene, often parallel to, or staying the same distance from, the subject. Some tripods attach to wheels (dollies) for smooth tracking. Shopping trolleys or wheelchairs are effective alternatives.

Moving camera work has become more acceptable with the increased use of news camcorders. It creates a true-to-life feel but is hard to do well with lightweight camcorders. Any camera movement is a special effect, so do not overdo it.

## EDITING GRAMMAR

Video editing is the process of putting together a sequence of moving pictures and sound. The purpose is to communicate information clearly to the audience. The editor directs attention by combining images so that the storyline unfolds consistently and coherently.

Video editing is an art that takes considerable practice to master fully, but the basic principles are quite simple. Editing grammar defines how to combine shots logically. The aim is to maintain continuity so that the editing process is unnoticed by the viewer. Following the rules of editing grammar results in effective image sequences and avoids common errors.

### The editing process

The editing process is one of selection and elimination. Each shot must have a purpose for it to be included. Ideally, only images that are essential to the narrative are used, and meaning is conveyed in a minimum number of shots.

### Shot sequences

The basic unit of video language is the shot sequence. A sequence is a number of connected shots that together create an impression, represent an event, tell a story or communicate an idea.

Usually a sequence begins with one or two long-shots to establish the location. They are followed by a mid-shot that focuses the area of interest within the wider scene. The remainder of the sequence is in close-up, concentrating the audience on details of the action or interaction. If the area of interest within the

Long-Shot (L.S.)

Mid-Shot (M.S.)

Close-Up. (C.U.)

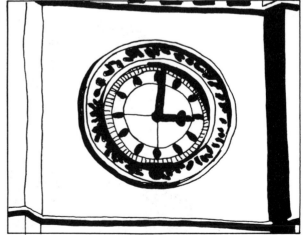

*Figure 9.11a* Shot sizes for (a) objects and (b) people

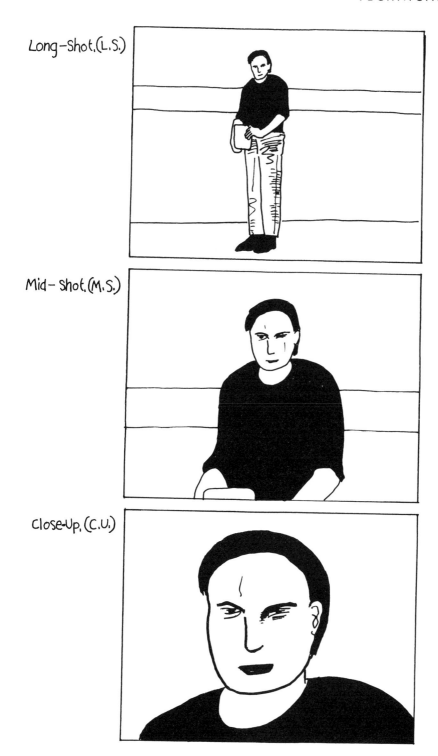

*Figure 9.11b*

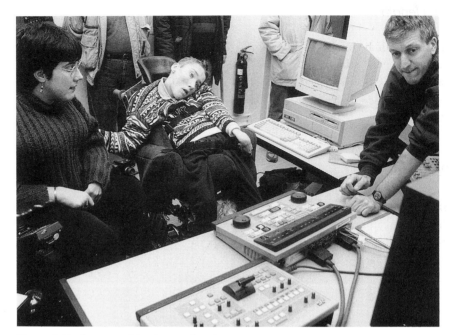

*Figure 9.12* Group working in an edit suite

wider scene changes, a mid-shot is used before more close-ups.

This standard pattern is followed in both drama and documentary. It is changed only for effect: for instance, starting close up, and only later drawing back to reveal the setting, creates suspense.

## Compressing time

One of the major reasons for editing is to compress time. If the representation of an event takes as long as the actual incident the viewer's interest is not sustained (at least in western culture). It is necessary to show only enough for the audience to take in what has happened. For instance, if a character travels from A to B, footage of the entire journey is not needed. Adequate illustration is provided by seeing them leaving, briefly during the journey, and arriving, possibly using a mileage signpost to show the journey length.

## Shot length

A shot should be long enough for the viewer to take in its purpose and meaning, but no longer. Beginners are often tempted to prolong shots. The exact length of each shot depends on the pace of the sequence and the feeling desired. However, 2–3 seconds is usually sufficient for a still shot, and 5–10 seconds for one containing movement; 15–20 seconds is plenty for a talking head.

## Pacing

Shot length and sequence rhythm contribute to the pacing of a programme and the impression it establishes. Regardless of the subject, the more cuts there are the faster the pacing, the shorter the programme seems, and the more interest it creates.

## Cutting visuals

Good editing is seamless. Cuts from one image to the next are invisible because they happen at moments when the audience is naturally ready to see the next shot.

To compress time and stimulate interest through constantly changing visuals, whilst giving the impression of a unbroken flow of images, a number of techniques are used.

## Insert shots

Insert shots show a central part of the action in close-up to concentrate the viewer on something important: for instance, in a detective drama, the cut to a hand hiding that vital piece of evidence.

## Cut-aways

Cut-away shots cut from the action to something or somewhere else. They are vital to creating continuity when compressing or expanding time. For instance, they are used to cover the visual jump caused by editing together two different sections of an interview (see jump cut below). Cut-aways should show something connected to the subject, or at least something that seems relevant.

## Points of view

One of the great things about communicating on video compared to, say, through theatre, is that the audience can be shown the action from a range of perspectives. In the theatre, the audience watches the whole play from one position. In a video, they may be presented with views from the front, the side, above, below, far away or close up. Frequently, a comment or action is followed by another character's reaction to it. This technique is used to define relationships and bring out emotions.

## Parallel action

Editing aims to get across maximum information, in an understandable form, in the minimum time. The more experiences provided, the more engaging the programme. Parallel editing is a technique used to develop two plots simultaneously by cutting back and forth between them.

# Breaking grammatical rules

There is a discontinuity in the smooth flow of images if the rules of editing grammar are broken.

## Jump cut

A jump cut occurs when the camera is switched off, and then switched on again without changing the shot. Some time has elapsed between one shot and the next, so people in the picture have changed position. The recording time discontinuity causes them to jump from place to place in the frame at the cut. Although this effect is deliberately created in the Disappearing Game, it is undesirable when editing.

It most commonly occurs when two soundbites from an interview are edited together, or when part of an event is cut out to compress time. It can also be produced if the same person appears in a different location in two consecutive shots, or if successive shots of two people are too similar in size and composition.

Jump cuts can be avoided in several ways:

- Consecutive shots show completely different people and places.
- A cut-away is inserted between the two shots (Figure 9.13).

- The angle to the subject and/or the size of shot changes considerably between one shot and the next.

## Crossing the line

Another common discontinuity is in direction of movement. The subject (person, car, ball) appears to be moving in one direction across the frame in one shot, and the opposite way in the next.

To avoid this, a line is visualized along the direction of movement. As long as the camera stays on the same side of the line from shot to shot, continuity of direction is maintained. If the camera crosses the line, the direction changes. Head-on shots and those from behind are neutral. To cut from one shot to another that has crossed the line, insert a neutral shot between them (Figure 9.14).

## Other jarring cuts

Editing mid-action always looks odd. Let the movement finish before cutting to the next shot.

Edits also jar if the shot does not make sense in the context. Every shot should be used for a reason.

## TEACHING IN PRACTICE

To provide a link between video operation and technical teaching this section illustrates how the teaching approach is put into practice.

Basic equipment operation is taught to every individual on a one-to-one basis as they take turns. They progress through repeated practice, the technical worker providing support, feedback and extra facts to refine their skills.

The first time an individual uses a piece of equipment, facilitate their learning by getting them to go through each step in a logical order. This establishes an operational procedure with them. Follow this procedure every time you work with them so that they learn through repeating the action. For example, camera operation can be taught as detailed below.

### Teaching camera operation

Get the camera operator to sit or stand behind the camera and take the lens cap off. This requires them to do something practical straight away.

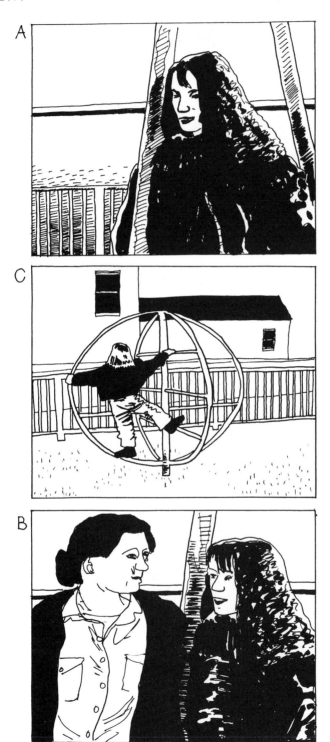

*Figure 9.13* Cut-away Shot C recorded between Shot A and Shot B to avoid jump cut

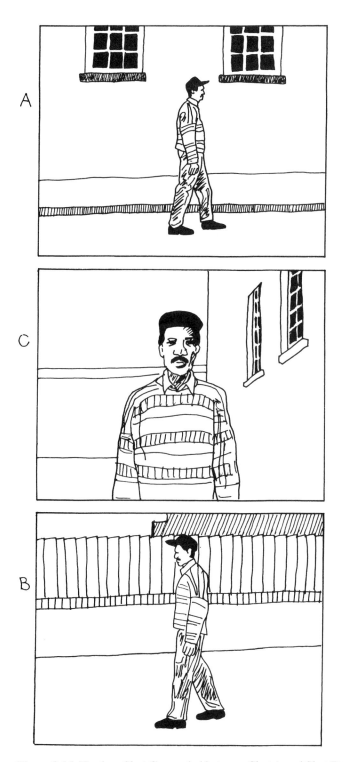

*Figure 9.14* Head-on Shot C recorded between Shot A and Shot B to avoid crossing the line

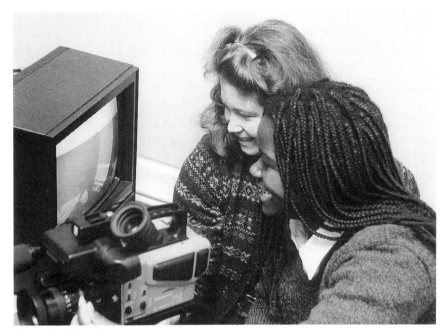

*Figure 9.15* Teaching camera operation

Show them the image on the viewfinder and on the monitor. Tell them to watch the monitor as it is larger and easier to see. If the individual is particularly intimidated, it may be hard for them to take anything in. Ask them what they can see on the monitor, to direct their concentration, and help by pointing things out. If the individual is fiddling with the equipment and not listening, encourage them to stand back, direct their attention to the monitor, and engage them by asking questions.

## Moving the camera

Next instruct them to hold the tripod arm, loosen the tripod, and practise moving the camera around to get different people in the picture. This establishes their contact with the equipment and places it in their control. If an individual is intimidated, you may have to place their hand on the tripod. Encourage them to move the camera by asking them to point at particular people or objects.

If the camera operator lets go of the tripod arm when it is loose, the camera can tip over, so watch carefully and remind them to keep hold if they look as though they might take their hand away. However, do not leap to the rescue unless the camera is in real danger. They need to learn the consequence of their actions.

## Focusing

Next get them to focus the camera. Ask them to point the camera at the subject. When working in the workshop situation, with the group sitting in a semi-circle, they can focus on any of the participants, as they are all the same distance from the camera. Indicate the zoom lever and invite them to try it out. Instruct them to move it until the person in front is as big as possible on the monitor. Make sure they move the zoom as far as it will go even if they can see only part of the person's face.

Ask them to turn the focus ring and point out how the picture goes clear and fuzzy. Tell them to make the picture as clear as possible. Support them by indicating if they are turning the ring too fast or the wrong way.

## Framing

When the picture is in focus, request that they move the zoom to frame the shot. Initially, help them decide on a shot size but do not worry too much as long as the person speaking is in the picture. Later, encourage them to frame on their own and help them to think more critically.

If the shot is stationary, ask them to tighten the tripod. If they are going to have to move the camera, ensure they keep it loose enough to pan and tilt smoothly.

## Recording

Finally, show them the on-off switch, and tell them to switch on after the floor manager counts in. Make sure that they press the switch firmly, and that recording has started. Stay with them during recording for support. Instruct them to make adjustments to the camera if necessary.

## After recording

Get them to switch off at the end. Then ensure that they tighten the tripod and put the lens cap on before replaying.

## *Pace*

With some practice this process is not too time-consuming. Even if time is short, create a sense of relaxation by your manner so that the camera operator does not feel rushed. The activity leader helps by keeping the rest of the group occupied.

## Progression

The second time an individual uses a piece of equipment, go through the same process reminding them of each step in the procedure, whilst reassuring them that it is normal to need reminding.

As time goes on they will become more self-sufficient. Let them work things out for themselves, but be there to support them if they are stuck. Do not be critical if they need full instruction each time.

Gather feedback on their understanding by asking them to describe what they are doing, and give new information to improve their work as appropriate.

# Teaching checklist

- Teach technical procedures through practice rather than theory.
- Set up activities that maximize hands-on experience with the equipment.
- Provide a framework that widens technical knowledge and develops skills over time.
- Start simply and introduce new operations only when relevant and contextualized.
- Let the participants set the pace. Provide new information only when they are ready.
- Give everyone some experience with the recording process before working on technical improvements. Allow them to make mistakes and learn through experience.
- Ask questions to assess the group's critical awareness.
- Do not make assumptions about technical abilities.
- Be encouraging and use positive criticism to reinforce confidence.
- Teach technical procedures on a one-to-one basis and promote equality of opportunity within the group.
- Remember that there may be different levels within the group. Be flexible and responsive to individual needs.
- Take time to answer questions but do not let the quicker participants set the pace or monopolize the workers' time.
- Teach without touching the equipment yourself, and do not demonstrate.
- Establish consistent operational procedures. Support individuals using the equipment, reinforcing skills through repetition.
- Do not use overly technical language or jargon. Use clear language to demystify the techniques.

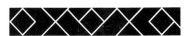

- Practise using the equipment until you are confident.
- Don't be too precious about the equipment. Trust the participants to take responsibility for it themselves.
- Know when to intervene to keep the equipment safe. In particular, be alert and ready to supervise when the camera is attached to the tripod, when the equipment is moved about, and to make sure that the lens cap is removed only when the camera is pointing away from the sun.

# Putting it into practice

Process is a term that connotes naturalness, an unfolding. . . . Method, on the other hand, implies a set of artificially created procedures. The terms go together because conceptions of processes are necessary to design methods to intervene in them – to encourage, guide, stop, or re-direct the processes.

(Brager and Specht 1975: 165)

This book has described a comprehensive methodology for using video with groups. Participatory video practice, however, like most group development work, is essentially an intuitive process rather than a rigid technique. The book covers the principles behind effective video usage and emphasizes the mistakes to avoid. It outlines practical activities and examples. Nevertheless, understanding remains theoretical until the techniques suggested are put into practice, and becoming skilled in the approach will take time.

This then is the starting point. The only way to develop full competence is to start working with a group to develop experience. The structure provided will guide you through the process, with an awareness of the potential problems, but specifically what is done at any stage will depend on the situation.

People are often more concerned about operating the equipment than facilitating group work. Remember that you do not need to be an expert. As long as you know the basics, and appreciate that genuine proficiency comes with practice, your production skills will grow working alongside the group. In fact, the real expertise needed to run a video project lies in flexible and appropriate group facilitation rather than video production. If the work is approached from the right perspective, the participants will benefit.

As each group is a unique collection of individuals, what works with one group may not work with the next. By becoming a reflective worker, prepared to learn from experience, by assessing what happened and why, your work will evolve and flourish. The participatory video approach responds to the specific situation and creates the opportunity for every participant to realize new capabilities and potential, so that both they and you are certain to find the work meaningful, exciting and inspiring.

# Appendix

Training and consultancy in participatory video is offered by:

REAL TIME VIDEO

Arts and Media Centre
21 South Street
Reading
Berks RG1 4QU

# Bibliography

Armes, R. (1988) *On Video*, London: Routledge.

Atienza, L. (1977) *VTR Workshop: Small Format Video*, Paris: UNESCO.

Biddle, W. and Biddle, L. (1966) *The Community Development Process, the Rediscovery of Local Initiative*, London: Holt, Rinehart & Winston.

Brager, G. and Specht, H. (1975) 'The process of community work' in R.M. Kramer and H. Specht (eds) *Readings in Community Organisation Practice*, New Jersey: Prentice-Hall.

Brandes, D. and Phillips, H. (1977) *Gamesters' Handbook*, Cheltenham: Stanley Thornes.

Brown, A. (1986) *Groupwork*, Aldershot: Gower.

Central Statistical Office (1995) *Social Trends 25*, London: HMSO.

Corrêa da Silva, H.B. (1988) 'Media for rural people's development' unpublished MSc Dissertation, University of Reading.

Dewey, J. (1949) *Experience and Education*, New York: Macmillan.

Douglas, T. (1976) *Groupwork Practice*, London: Tavistock.

Dowmunt, T. (1987) *Video with Young People*, London: Cassell/Inter-Action in Print.

Friere, P. (1972) *Pedagogy of the Oppressed*, New York: Herder & Herder.

Gerbner, G. and Gross, L. (1976) 'Living with television: the violence profile', *Journal of Communication* 28: 3.

Hénaut, D. (1971) 'Powerful catalyst', *Challenge for Change Newsletter* 7, Montreal.

——— (1975) 'Asking the right questions: video in the hands of the citizens (the challenge for change experience)', speech given at an international conference in Australia.

Lewis, J. (1991) *The Ideological Octopus*, New York: Routledge.

Liebmann, M. (1986) *Art Therapy for Groups: A Handbook of Themes, Games and Exercises*, London: Routledge.

McLellan, I. (1987) 'Video and narrowcasting: TV for and by ordinary people', *Rural Development* December 20 (4).

Mander, J. (1978) *Four Arguments for the Elimination of Television*, New York: William Morrow.

Redl, F. (1951) 'Art of group composition' in S. Shulze (ed.) *Creative Living in a Children's Institution*, New York: Association Press.

Report of the National Enquiry in the Arts (1992) *Arts and Communities*, London: Community Development Foundation.

Shaw, J. (1986) 'Process work and community video practice', *Independent Media* 57.

——— (1992) 'Real time, real issues', *Mailout* June.

Srinivasan, L. (1992) *Options for Educators: A Monograph for Decision Makers on Alternative Participatory Strategies*, New York: PACT/CDS.

Stewart, S. (1988) 'Video as a tool in training and organising', *VITA News* July/Oct.

Stuart, M. (1981) 'Village solutions make global community', *Inter Media* September.

Wade, G. (1980) *Street Video*, Leicester: Blackthorne Press.

# Index